NEUROBIOLOGY OF ALCOHOL ABUSE

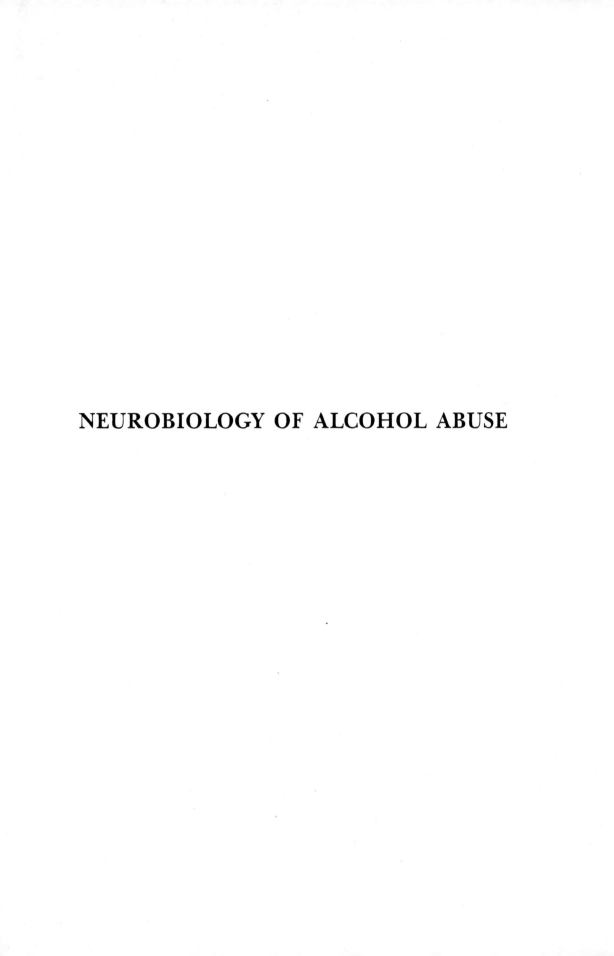

The five volumes in this series are:

1. *Alcoholism: Its Natural History, Chemistry and General Metabolism.*
2. *The Neurobiology of Alcohol Abuse.*
3. *The Psychodynamics of Alcoholism: A Current Synthesis.*
4. *Alcoholism and Women, Genetics, Fetal Development, and Polydrug Abuse.*
5. *Alcoholism, Co-Dependency, Recovery and the Role of the Clinician.*

NEUROBIOLOGY OF ALCOHOL ABUSE

By

WILLIAM J. HAUGEN LIGHT, Ph.D.

Institute for the Study of Drugs,
Alcohol, and Addictive Behaviors

and

Department of Biology
Metropolitan State College

Graduate School of Public Affairs
University of Colorado at Denver

Research Associate
California Academy of Sciences

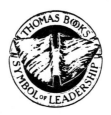

CHARLES C THOMAS • PUBLISHER
Springfield • Illinois • U.S.A.

Published and Distributed Throughout the World by

CHARLES C THOMAS • PUBLISHER
2600 South First Street
Springfield, Illinois 62717

© *1986 by* CHARLES C THOMAS • PUBLISHER

ISBN 0-398-05197-6

Library of Congress Catalog Card Number: 85-20883

Printed in the United States of America
SC-R-3

Library of Congress Cataloging in Publication Data

Light, William J. Haugen.
    Neurobiology of alcohol abuse.

    Bibliography: p.
    Includes index.
    1. Nervous system—Diseases. 2. Alcohol—Toxicology.
3. Alcoholism. 4. Alcoholism—Complications and
sequelae. I. Title. [DNLM: 1. Alcoholism.
2. Neurophysiology. WM 274 L723n]
RC346.L49 1986   616.86′1   85-20883
ISBN 0-398-05197-6

To the Muellers:
Carl and Mimi, and Marc, Eric and Dierdre;
good friends, fine relatives and wonderful people.

PREFACE

This series of volumes is written as an introduction to the complex and often bewildering illness of alcoholism. It is directed primarily to health care professionals, particularly medical students, practicing physicians, psychiatric and psychological clinicians and trainees, nurses, alcoholism counselors, and other practitioners who regularly confront alcoholism as either the primary illness or as a major complicating factor in their patients or clients. One may legitimately ask, why another series on alcoholism? They seem to be coming off the presses at a brisk rate already from nearly every quarter—as though another new fad has burst upon us and one is not really "with it" unless one is either a recovered alcoholic intent upon telling his or her own story, or else is involved in treating them in some way. One can scarcely keep up with the literature in one's own specialty, let alone the proliferation of books and articles about alcoholism. Why burden us with yet more?

My response is that the works currently available overwhelmingly treat the subject from the fairly narrow perspective in which the authors or editors are themselves research experts, or out of the need to advance a favorite model or theory about the cause(s), course and preferred treatment of the problem. Or if they are more general and ecclectic in scope, the discussion is far too superficial to be of any real value for professional workers who wish to know the current state of our knowledge of "ethanology." The last ten years or so have seen an enormous growth in our understanding about alcohol and alcoholism research. At some point in the very recent past we acquired a critical mass of accurate, scientific information about the pharmacological mechanisms by which alcohol (and many other addictive agents, as well) affects membrane systems and leads to pharmacological tolerance and physical dependence. These data, coupled with an increasingly sophisticated understanding of the psychodynamic and biochemical factors contributing to psychiatric illness in general and our ability to effectively intervene in such illnesses to an unprecedented degree, have permitted an understanding of alcoholic disorders at a most fundamental level—a level that rivals our comprehension of our world and our universe in the other cognate sciences.

This information, unfortunately, is widely scattered in numerous professional journals and symposium volumes in the fields of medicine, toxicology and pharmacology, physiology, psychiatry and psychology. It is also heavily burdened with highly technical jargon and it assumes a command of the relevant background literature that is rarely possessed by anyone not actively working in the research frontiers of the respective discipline. These comments also apply to recent reviews on the subject (for example, Lieber 1982).

It was my intention to bring together the substance of this vast literature, organize it into what I hope is a holistic and coherent picture, and translate it into comprehensible English that can be readily understood by any reasonably intelligent and educated person. I am convinced that this can be accomplished without sacrificing any of the scientific accuracy or subtle nuances of understanding to be obtained from close attention to the fine details and interrelationships of the various systems involved.

Thus, an adequate comprehension of the many factors contributing to alcoholic liver disease requires a detailed knowledge of liver structure and function. It is especially important to know how the structural units of the liver typically described in medical texts correlate with the physiologically more useful "functional" hepatic units, the liver acini, and how their concentric zones of increasing anoxia toward the perivenular areas lead to specific regional hepatic lesions, necrosis, and ultimately, fibrosis. One must also be aware of the biochemical details of the mixed-function monooxygenases (which are only now beginning to be adequately taught in medical schools), basic pharmacokinetics and enzymatic processes, general lipid metabolism, the involvement of the pituitary-adrenal axis and catecholamine release upon peripheral free fatty acid mobilization, and the bewildering array of metabolic consequences of altered redox states resulting from alcohol oxidation.

This series is meant to be a current synthesis of information from many different fields and an examination of the disease of alcoholism as I have come to know it over nearly seventeen years of professional study. It is based, among other things, upon my experience in working with alcoholics and their families as supervising counselor for the National Council on Alcoholism in the San Francisco Bay area. It incorporates a background and education spanning many years as a professional scientist and educator and which includes formal training in toxicology at the University of Wisconsin at Madison. It grew out of a series of lectures that I developed for a wide range of audiences, ranging from youngsters on probation for alcohol and drug related offenses, through volunteer workers and counselor-trainees in alcohol intervention, to formal classes of nursing and medical students at the University of San Francisco and the University of California School of Medicine at San Francisco, and finally, both undergraduate and graduate level courses in pharmacology of addictions at Metropolitan State College and the University of Colorado, both schools in Denver.

Although I have assumed no particular background or professional training on the part of the readers, it is expected that they have at least some basic understanding of the nature of chemical bonds and can comprehend the simple structural formulae presented herein. Those with absolutely no understanding of these concepts are referred to the chapters on the chemistry of life to be found in any good biology textbook. These subjects are also discussed more fully in the first volume of this series (Light 1985).

Some readers will perhaps have psychological foundations, some medical, some may be members of the clergy, some paraprofessional counselors of various persuasions with or without formal scientific training, and some may be interested laypersons who are themselves recovering or recovered alcoholics or the close friends and significant others of alcoholics. Because of the disparate backgrounds of the readership to which this series of books is directed, I have introduced each topic with a basic examination of the terminology and processes under discussion. The reader is led step by step through ever more advanced and sophisticated concepts up to and including the latest information, ideas, and thinking entertained by current researchers in the field.

Therefore, a family practice or general physician may be initially annoyed at elementary discussions of such things as oxidation-reduction reactions. These are included, however, so that someone from another discipline, let us say clinical psychology, will be able to follow subsequent treatments of the metabolic significance of altered redox states consequent to the oxidation of large amounts of alcohol and the ultimate effects of these processes upon human cognition and behavior.

The medically or biologically sophisticated reader will soon enough encounter very detailed presentations of biochemical phenomena that are currently at the forefronts of scientific investigation—subjects that will most certainly not have been studied if he or she has been in practice for even a very few years (like less than five or six). Indeed, many of these subjects have yet to be incorporated into standard medical texts or curricula. At the same time, our clinical psychologist will have been educated up to the level of the medical or research professional, at least insofar as is immediately relevant to a full understanding of the topic under consideration. Elsewhere the situation will be reversed, so that it is now the psychiatrically erudite reader who must tolerate the initial, elementary presentation of such things as depressive-spectrum disorder, sociopathy and its relationship to primary and secondary alcoholism and the rudimentary concepts of decompensation and regression, narcissistic trauma and entitlement loss. But here, too, the discussion will soon lead into such topics as the interrelationship between narcissism and paranoid ideation in alcoholics, dyadic versus triadic conflicts, and the relative degrees of bonding and socialization in the development of the psychoses, neuroses and personality disorders. The latest concepts involving imbalances of central neurotransmitter substances as major factors in psychiatric disturbances, including alcoholism, are explored in depth and fully integrated with more traditional psychodynamic models. I believe this series represents the only work to date that truly accomplishes this goal in a fundamental and coherent way.

I am introducing a number of ideas of my own about alcoholism which are presented for the first time in this series of volumes. I do have personal biases about this disorder, as does anyone who has thought about it seriously for more than ten minutes. Some of these ideas conflict with certain theories of some other authors. This is most evident in the portions dealing with the etiological factors underlying alcoholism, a subject which has spawned much often acrimonious debate. However, my suggestions are quite in line with the medical and psychiatric consensus about alcoholic disorders, and they are thoughts to which I have given careful consideration and brought wide-ranging knowledge and experience. I cannot prove some of these ideas, but I think they are as valid as anyone's. They are based upon personal insight and understanding, both intuitive and scientifically objective, of the various dynamics involved. They are certainly no more flimsily grounded than is most of the clinical and psychiatric literature, which is similarly anecdotal. The major portion of this work is, of course, firmly based upon solidly demonstrated, scientific data—particularly those sections dealing with the pharmacological and biological aspects of alcoholism.

Although much of the material contained in these volumes is difficult and complex, it is presented in what I hope is an easy, communicative, and readable style. I have provided a great many graphic illustrations to aid the users of these books, and innumerable footnotes supply additional information to enhance a point or to correlate the discussion with other related phenomena. I have not encumbered the text with extensive citations from the professional literature. This information is in the public domain and is well documented by the references which I do include. This series is also not intended to be an exhaustive, encyclopaedic catalog of facts and statistics about alcoholism. Rather, it attempts to provide a comprehensive and holistic synthesis of the many interrelated psychodynamic and biological processes which contribute to the etiology and manifestations of alcoholic disorders. The information contained herein is the product of a huge army of investigators and clinicians in many fields whose work spans many decades. I have served primarily as an interpreter.

I have covered little of the ground previously discussed for general audiences by other authors, although some review of such information is appropriate and is included. An example is a detailed presentation of the course of primary alcoholism as originally described by the late Dr. E. M. Jellinek. But even here, the discussion has been modernized and tempered with a much wider clinical experience than was available in Jellinek's time. And a few qualifying remarks of my own are included. I will not go very deeply into the various debates on treatment modalities, although I will present a broad approach based upon the overwhelming medical and psychiatric consensus in the final volume of this series. And I do not propose to engage in the endless debate about whether alcoholics can safely return to drinking on a social basis. I will categorically state my firm conviction that they cannot, and that any attempt to suggest that they can is medically and psychiatrically irresponsible. As to the sections dealing with the pharmacology, toxicology and metabolism of alcohol, and the genetics, biology, natural history and medical aspects of alcoholism, my discussions are confined to hard, scientifically verifiable facts and interpretations, and any inferences I may draw are based upon these hard data and are also supported in the professional literature.

I had originally intended to write a book for the recovering alcoholic and his or her family, inasmuch as many of them, regardless of the particular treatment modality in which they may be participating, are largely ignorant about the disease, its causes, course, and medical and psychological consequences (as are the great majority of health care professionals). Although many alcoholics make full recoveries and are able to lead rich and satisfying lives, many others are plagued by recurrent or chronic depressions of profound proportions and are afflicted by a variety of physical and emotional problems that require professional intervention—a form of assistance they all too rarely get.

But as the manuscript progressed it became apparent that I was getting far too deep into the scientific details and complexities of the alcoholic disorders to keep the attention of most laypersons for long. This was obviously the case despite my efforts to make it palatable to a wide range of readers and clearly understandable by any fairly intelligent and literate person willing to put in the necessary effort. About this time my wife, who is a practicing physician, suggested that I was actually writing for a professional audience and that I should continue in that genre. She observed that a much less detailed synopsis of this work would be more appropriate for the average reader.

What I have done in this series is to provide a thorough and detailed introduction into each discipline so that nonspecialists will understand the many intricacies of normal function of each system under consideration. Thus, the volume dealing with the effects of alcohol and alcoholism upon the human nervous system begins with a review of basic neurobiology. One has to know how neurons function and transmit information before one can appreciate how alcohol affects those processes. Similarly, one cannot really appreciate the ways in which alcohol ravages embryonic development or understand fetal alcohol syndrome without some basic knowledge of normal human fetal development. So each topic is presented as a detailed minicourse for those who know little or nothing about it. This is true of the psychodynamics volumes as well as the biologically and medically oriented ones. Following the introductory sections, the effects of alcohol and alcohol abuse upon the respective systems are presented in great detail. And a summary is provided at the end of each section for those without the heart or inclination to wade through all the heavy scientific material. Certain fundamental biochemical concepts discussed in Volume 1 of this series (Light 1985) are not repeated in the later volumes, and the reader is referred to that volume if clarification is required.

This series of volumes presents, I believe, as complete an integrated a picture of alcoholism as it is currently possible to create. And I think the model described in this series is a powerful and useful one. Alcoholism, perhaps more than most psychiatric disorders, can be understood at several fundamental levels. This series of books is my contribution to that end.

This work took four years to complete, and the final manuscript was more than one thousand pages and a quarter of a million words in length. There were some 90 full page illustrations. Because of the enormous cost of producing a single or even two-volume book from this manuscript, costs which would have priced this work far beyond the reach of most of us (including myself), the publisher and I agreed to present this as a series of five volumes, each about two hundred or so pages long. To fully grasp the entire picture requires all five of these volumes. Nevertheless, each one is self-contained and presents a complete picture of alcoholism and the respective topics contained therein.

I, at least, have grown enormously both professionally and personally by writing this series. It has enabled me to provide my students at the Institute for the Study of Drugs, Alcohol and Addictive Behaviors at Metropolitan State College and the University of Colorado at Denver with extraordinarily valuable information and insight to take with them into the world of addiction prevention, intervention, treatment, and education.

W. J. H. L.

Colorado Springs
August 12, 1985

ACKNOWLEDGMENTS

I owe an enormous debt to many individuals, organizations and institutions who made this series possible. Among these are: Mrs. Florette White Pomeroy, retired executive director of the National Council on Alcoholism—Bay Area, who gave me free rein during my tenure there and staunchly supported my sometimes unusual methods of intervention; Dr. Mary Fortin, formerly of the School of Nursing at the University of San Francisco; Dr. Mark I. Levy, a loyal companion in a common cause who walked an enormous distance with me along the incredible path of discovery and enlightenment; Dr. Anotonio J. Ferreira, who freely shared many of his keen insights with me deriving from his private psychiatric practice focusing on alcoholics and their families; Mr. Mitch Capor of the Alameda County Probation Department, California, who provided an ongoing opportunity to gain valuable insight into the special problems of teenage substance abuse; my wife, Dr. Ruth Lewert Light, who has been a constant source of strength and inspiration throughout both our lives together and the writing of this manuscript; and my students in introductory and advanced courses in pharmacology and psychodynamics of addictions at the Institute for the Study of Drugs, Alcohol, and Addictive Behaviors at both Metropolitan State College and the University of Colorado at Denver, who forced me to continually consolidate, sharpen and refine my thoughts about the subject and who always remind me of my vast ignorance.

Words cannot express my deep gratitude to the many thousands of men and women in Alcoholics Anonymous and its sister fellowship, Al-Anon. Perhaps this series of volumes may be regarded as a small repayment for all the pain and joy that they have shared with me and for the many lifetime friendships that have sprung up between us. This work is for them, the recovered and recovering alcoholics and co-alcoholics, who have shown the way to so many thousands of suffering victims of this most horrible of afflictions.

Finally, I thank Drs. John J. Magnuson and Ronald D. Hinsdill of the

University of Wisconsin at Madison, who provided more than they know, who good naturedly tolerated my eccentricities, and who generously allowed me to wear both my hats simultaneously. The writing of this manuscript was supported in part by the Department of Health and Human Services Public Health Service National Research Award 5 T32 ES07015 to the University of Wisconsin from the National Institute of Environmental Health Sciences.

LIST OF FIGURES

CONTENTS

NEUROBIOLOGY OF ALCOHOL ABUSE

INTRODUCTION TO NEUROBIOLOGY

The structural units of the nervous system are the nerve cells or *neurons* and the various supporting, nurturing and protective *glial cells* collectively known as *neuroglia*. The neuron is highly specialized for the generation and transmission of nervous impulses. It contains most of the usual organelles and ultrastructural features common to all animal cells. In addition, it has a number of structural features not found in other cell types (figure 1). The *cell body* or *soma* contains the DNA-bearing nucleus and usually only one *nucleolus*—a smaller dark-staining body lacking an enveloping membrane which consists of *ribosomal RNA* and proteins and which is involved in the production of the rRNA-protein subunits which are assembled into ribosomes in the cytoplasm. The ribosomes are responsible for the synthesis of proteins.[1] The cell body of the neuron also contains dense aggregations of ribosomal rough endoplasmic reticulum known as *Nissl bodies* which continuously replace the proteins used by the various functions of the neuron. These proteins are packaged up in glyco- or lipoprotein envelopes by the Golgi apparatus and transported to the distal portions of the cell.

One or more elongated cell processes sprout from the neuronal cell body. *Dendrites* are fibers of varying length which carry nervous impulses toward the cell body. Processes and conducting structures of various kinds which carry impulses or substances toward the central portion of a

---

[1]The reader is referred to Volume 1 of this series for more detail about these structures (Light 1985). The nuclear DNA serves as a coded template from which a "negative" sequence of 3-base "words" or *codons* is synthesized into *messenger RNA*. *Bases* are nitrogen-containing subunits of the nucleotides which form DNA—the codon triplets which they form constitute the basis of the genetic code which decrees the exact sequence in which amino acids will come together to create specific proteins. The mRNA negative synthesized from the DNA template then moves out of the nucleus into the cytoplasm where it enters the ribosomes in a zipper-like fashion. Meanwhile, *transfer RNA* units within the cytoplasm recognize and attach to specific amino acids depending upon the specific end groups. These tRNA-amino acid complexes bear specific 3-base reciprocal *anticodons* which are attracted to and join the corresponding codon exposed in the ribosomal "zipper" as the mRNA is passed through. As each tRNA anticodon connects to the mRNA codon, the amino acid is joined to the end of a growing protein chain by a *peptide bond*. (See also Volume 4 of this series.)

cell, system, or the organism as a whole are described by the adjective *afferent* (this descriptor applies to blood vessels as well as nerve fibers).[2] Dendrites typically communicate with thousands of other neurons at highly specialized junctions called *synapses.* The dendrites carry impulses from these other neurons and pass them on to those farther along in the chain of propagation.

Axons are single fibers, one per neuron, which emerge from the cell body and which carry impulses down the line from the soma—they are thus the *efferent* part of the nerve cell.[2] Axons frequently have one or more collateral branches that connect with other neurons or end organs. These collaterals often function in various regulatory feed-back loops, especially within the CNS, as we shall see shortly.

Axons may be either *myelinated* or *nonmyelinated* and both types are widely distributed throughout both the central and peripheral nervous systems. Myelinated axons are enveloped in a concentric series of double membranes formed by specialized cells adjacent to the neuron which wrap around the axon many times (figure 2). Such *myelin sheaths* around peripheral axons are formed by *Schwann cells* and the outer membrane is called the *neurilemma.* Within the central nervous system itself there are no Schwann cells and the myelin sheaths are formed out of specialized glial cells known as *oligodendrocytes* (figure 2). Peripheral Schwann cells wrap many times around a single axon, or they may carry a number of nonmyelinated axons, each lying within an invagination of the neurilemma. Such bundles of nonmyelinated axons lying within a single Schwann cell are known as *Remak bundles* (figure 2). Within the central nervous system each oligodendrocyte forms tight multiple spirals around several axons in a manner very similar to the way in which Schwann cells wrap around a single axon. Regions densely packed with myelinated, white-colored fibers within the CNS are collectively called the *white matter* of the brain or spinal cord. Similarly, regions consisting mostly of the nonmyelinated cell bodies and dendrites of those same fibers, along with neuroglia, are called the *gray matter.*[3]

Within the peripheral nervous system the myelin sheaths are not

---

[2]These terms also apply to entire neurons or pathways of several neurons. For example, nerve fibers bringing signals into the central nervous system (spinal cord and/or the brain) are afferent fibers. Those carrying messages out to the periphery of the organism (for example, commands to certain muscle groups to react in a given way) are called efferent fibers.

[3]In preserved brain material these regions are hard and gray. In living brains this portion is typically soft and pinkish-brown.

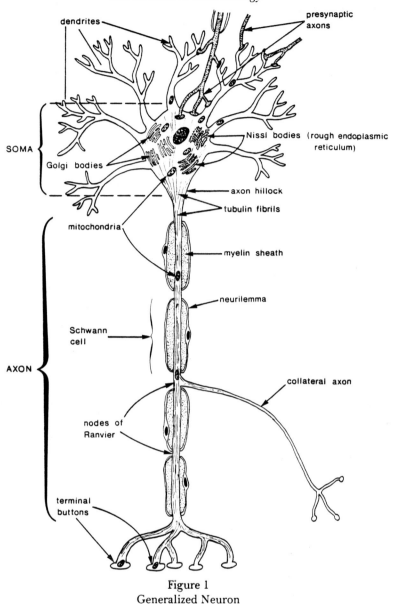

Figure 1
Generalized Neuron

continuous along the lengths of their enclosed axons. Instead they are interrupted at periodic, more or less even intervals by short gaps where the axons are in direct contact with the extracellular medium. These gaps are called the *nodes of Ranvier* (figure 1) and they are vital to the rapid conduction of nervous impulses over long distances, a process to be described shortly. Each segment of myelin sheath between two adjacent nodes of Ranvier represents a single Schwann cell.

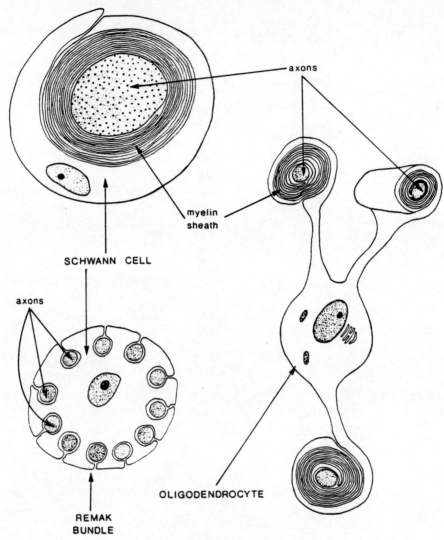

Figure 2
Patterns of Myelination

Redrawn from Bowman & Rand 1980 and Warwick & Williams 1973, and slightly modified.

As is true for all animal cells, neurons are surrounded by a *plasma membrane.* Such membranes are composed of a double layer of *phospholipids*—molecules in which two fatty acids are linked to a glycerol molecule, while the third methylene group of the glycerol is occupied by a polar phosphate group (see Volume 1 of this series for discussions of these and other chemical phenomena; Light 1985). The polar phosphate heads of the phospholipids are readily attracted to the equally polar water molecules in the cellular and intercellular media, whereas the nonpolar fatty-acid tails are repelled by the water. This results in their spontaneous arrangement into two layers with the polar heads directed outwards toward the watery environment and the nonpolar, hydrophobic tails pointing inward. Scattered within this double-layered matrix (the *phospholipid bilayer*) are various globular proteins which function as enzymes, structural units, ionic gates and their receptors, or which serve as carrier molecules in the active or facilitated transport of other molecules across the membrane. This is illustrated in figure 3 (see also figure 23).

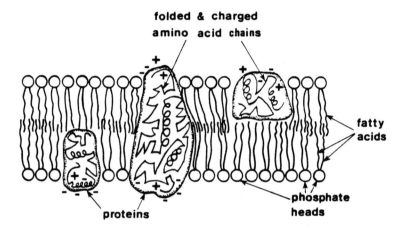

CELL MEMBRANE

Figure 3
Membrane Structure

Some idea of the manner in which a resting neuron maintains a constant difference in electric charge between the inside and outside of the neural membrane—the so-called *resting potential*—is critical to any understanding of how chemical agents affect human consciousness and behavior. This phenomenon is here presented in some detail.

In figure 4, the neuron is represented as a simple enclosed compartment separated from the extracellular environment by a selectively permeable membrane. All cellular processes borne by neurons in actuality are omitted from the diagram for the sake of clarity. As previously described, the cell membrane almost totally (but not quite) excludes sodium ions from diffusing down their concentration gradient into the neuron. On the other hand, potassium ions can migrate through the membrane quite freely, and they tend to flow down their concentration gradient to the exterior of the neuron by simple diffusion. The sodium-potassium pump continuously forces the K^+ back into the cell, however, in a process requiring the expenditure of much energy by converting ATP into ADP. The resulting concentration of Na^+ relative to the K^+ in the extracellular environment is about 10:1. Conversely, the concentration of K^+ relative to Na^+ inside the neuron is also about 10:1. The presence of large organic anions or negatively charged particles tends to exclude other, inorganic anions such as chloride (Cl^-) from entering the cell. The organic anions include such acids as aspartine and glutamate, which are far too large to move across the neural membrane. The exclusion of chloride ions from the neuron's interior is important in the generation of inhibitory potentials, as we shall see.

The resting potential of about -70 millivolts results from the fact that the sodium-potassium pump cannot quite keep pace with the constant leaking of K^+ to the exterior. Because of this slight deficit of positive ions inside the membrane relative to the outside (there are slightly more Na^+ outside than there are K^+ inside), a relative net minus charge exists inside the membrane. Figure 5 shows the operational details of the sodium-potassium pump. The carrier protein involved, Na^+-K^+—dependent ATPase, binds only to K^+ when the carrier is non-phosphorylated—that is, when no high-energy phosphate group is attached. Conversely, the carrier attaches only to Na^+ when the former is phosphorylated. On the inner membrane surface, the nonphosphorylated carrier is attached to a K^+ ion. In the presence of a magnesium-dependent *kinase* (a kinase is an enzyme which facilitates the movement of its protein substrate), ATP gives up one of its phosphates to the carrier protein, becoming converted into ADP in the process. The now phosphorylated carrier enzyme immediately gives up its K^+ and binds onto a Na^+. Furthermore, the absorbtion of the energy contained in the phosphate by the carrier, causes the carrier to move across to the outer surface of the neural membrane, perhaps by a rotational process. On the outer membrane surface, a second enzyme—*ATP-phosphatase*—causes the phosphate group to detach from the carrier protein. This causes the carrier to immediately give up its Na^+, which is then released into the extracellular medium, and to bind to one of the K^+ which has leaked to the outside. The resulting loss of energy contained in the phosphate group causes the carrier and its bound K^+ to move back across the membrane to

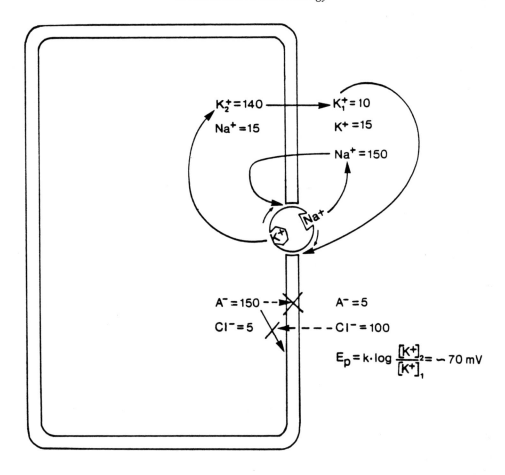

Figure 4
Schematic Model of the Resting Potential

The neural membrane is only slightly permeable to Na^+ which enters the cell in very small amounts by diffusion down its concentration gradient. The membrane is very highly permeable to K^+ which leak readily to the outside. Although the sodium-potassium pump rapidly transports the influxing Na^+ back to the cell's exterior and the leaked K^+ back into the cell, it cannot quite keep pace with the massive leakage of K^+ to the outside. This results in a net deficit of positive charge inside the membrane relative to the exterior ($K^+ = 140$ inside relative to $Na^+ = 150$ outside), generating a resting potential of about -70 millivolts. Discounting the leakage of K^+ through the membrane, the amounts of K^+ outside and of Na^+ inside the membrane are approximately equal and about an order of magnitude less than their respective concentrations on opposite sides of the membrane. Organic anions such as glutamate and aspartate are far too large to pass through the membrane pores, and their minus charges repel the tendency of Cl^- to flow into the cell down its concentration gradient. The modified Nernst equation shows the relationship between the inside ($[K^+]_2$) and outside ($[K^+]_1$) potassium ion concentrations (in mmol/l) and the electrostatic potential (E_p); k is a condensed constant incorporating several factors and is equal to 61. Dotted lines indicate blocked pathways. Modified from Bowman & Rand 1980.

the inner surface. At this point, the carrier is again phosphorylated, gives up its K^+ and accepts an Na^+, and the entire process is repeated.

Unlike most other cells which can also burn fats and amino acids as alternate fuels, neurons can utilize only glucose. And also unlike most other tissues, neurons cannot function anaerobically for even the shortest period. The brain is entirely dependent upon oxidative metabolism. Because of the need to maintain a constant resting potential across the neural membranes of each of the brain's more than 10^{11} (100 billion) nerve cells, the normal functioning of these neurons requires an enormous expenditure of both oxygen and glucose-derived energy. The total energy output of the brain due to the sodium-potassium pump does not vary much throughout the course of a day. The resting potential must be maintained regardless of the activity levels or state of consciousness of the organism, and this requires the continual operation of the sodium-potassium active transport pump. If the supply of either oxygen or glucose to the brain is interrupted, consciousness will be lost and permanent brain damage will occur *within ten seconds!*

THE NERVOUS IMPULSE

A nervous impulse is generated when an incoming stimulus causes the neural membrane to become suddenly very permeable to Na^+; these ions rush in through the membrane from the outside, resulting in a reversal of polarity with the inside of the membrane now positive relative to the outside. Figure 6 illustrates how a series of *graded impulses* traverse the cell body of the neuron. Graded impulses occur when incoming stimuli from other neurons reach the soma or cell body of the neuron under consideration. These impulses vary in strength with the strength of the stimulus and they are characterized by both *spatial* and *temporal summation*—that is, they are additive over distance and time. The stronger the stimulus, the stronger is the graded impulse, and the stronger the impulse, the greater the distance over which it is propagated before becoming attenuated and dying out (see the graded response graph in figure 6). Additionally, stronger stimuli produce a more rapid firing of graded impulses across the soma, and these repeated responses are summed over time and distance, resulting in a stronger combined impulse which lasts longer and travels farther. There is a slight swelling between the cell body of the neuron and the base of the axon known as the *axon hillock*. If the series of graded potentials generated across the

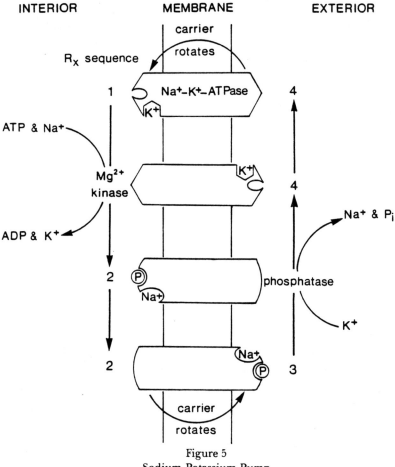

Figure 5
Sodium-Potassium Pump

Sodium and potassium ions are transported to the outer and inner surfaces of the cell membrane, respectively, by means of an ATP-driven carrier protein, Na^+-K^+-dependent ATPase. In the presence of Na^+ and divalent magnesium cation (Mg^{2+}-dependent kinase), the terminal phosphate is transferred from ATP to the carrier (1–2). Once the ATPase is phosphorylated it will bind to Na^+ but not to K^+. It thus gives up any K^+ it is carrying and binds to an intracellular sodium ion (2). The Na^+-bearing, phosphorylated carrier protein, being a large instrinsic membrane protein, undergoes a stereochemical transformation by which it transports the Na^+ across the width of the membrane to the outer surface, perhaps by a rotational process as figured above (3). Once on the outer surface of the membrane, the binding site on the carrier enzyme gives up the attached Na^+ in response to the presence of K^+ in the medium (3–4). In this process the carrier is dephosphorylated and the K^+ replaces the previously bound Na^+, which is now released into the extracellular medium (4). The dephosphorylated carrier is again stereochemically transformed so that it transports the K^+ across the cell membrane to the inner surface (4-1). Once inside the cell membrane (1), the binding site is again phosphorylated in the presence of intracellular sodium and magnesium, the K^+ is released, a new Na^+ taken up, and the entire process is repeated. In fact, there are multiple binding sites specific for Na^+ and for K^+ on each Na^+-K^+-ATPase molcular complex (Roach 1979).

soma reach the axon hillock with a combined intensity[4] equal to the required *threshold level*—a depolarization of about 15 millivolts smaller than the resting potential—a sweeping, all-or-none *action potential* is generated consisting of a self-propagating reversal in membrane potential that moves rapidly down the entire length of the axon. The details of graded potential initiation will be discussed shortly. It is first necessary to examine the nature of the action potential and the details of passing a nervous impulse from one neuron to another.

In nonmyelinated fibers, the sudden permeability of the membrane to Na^+ created by an action potential allows the sodium ions to rush inside the axon membrane creating a quick reversal in the membrane's polarity. This is due to the sudden addition of Na^+ ions to the already present K^+ ions, causing the inner surface of the membrane to become now strongly positive relative to the outside. This abrupt reversal of polarity in one small region of the axonal membrane causes the adjacent region down the path of propagation to become very permeable to Na^+ influx, resulting in a polarity reversal at this point, and so on down the line. The sudden increase in Na^+ permeability is due to the configurational changes in specific *channel proteins* or gates specific to given ions. As the gates undergo configuration changes in response to the perturbations of membrane electrostatic polarity, the previously barred ions can now enter freely.[5] Such an involved process by which the action potential in nonmyelinated fibers is induced section by consecutive section along an axon is relatively slow and inefficient as a means of propagation of a nervous impulse.

Transmission along a myelinated axon is quite another matter. In myelinated fibers the sodium-potassium interchange occurs only at the nodes of Ranvier (figure 7). Here there are two major effects of the depolarization: (1) an abrupt, but very brief increase in Na^+ permeability, and (2) a delayed, but longer lasting increase in K^+ permeability. A membrane depolarization of about 4 mV will produce a threefold increase in Na^+ permeability. The change in electric field alters the shape of

---

[4]Graded potentials can be either excitatory (additive) or inhibitory (subtractive). It is the sum total of all the additive and subtractive potentials at the axon hillock that determines whether an action potential will occur.

[5]Proteins carry a number of electric charges distributed at various sites along their lengths. These charges are quite specific and are the immediate consequence of the precise sequence of amino acids of which the proteins are constructed. Any alteration of the electrical charges in the membranes within which these proteins are embedded, will cause specific conformational changes in the proteins themselves (see also figure 23).

charged membrane proteins and specific sodium channels are opened. The Na$^+$ rushes inside down its concentration gradient, causing the membrane potential to reverse. The sodium gates close again very rapidly, and the Na$^+$ permeability of the membrane is extinguished almost as soon as it appears. The very brief duration of the Na$^+$ inrush coincides with the electrical spike of the action potential in that particular region (a given node of Ranvier)—a positive inside potential of 30 to 60 mV relative to the exterior.

At this point, the membrane becomes extremely permeable to K$^+$ (more so than usual), and it, too, moves down its concentration gradient and exits the cell at the node in question. This K$^+$ egress repolarizes the axon so that there is again a net negative charge on the inside relative to the outside. However, this polarity is due to an excess of K$^+$ on the outside relative to Na$^+$ on the inside. Since the propagation of a nervous impulse requires that sodium rush inward through suddenly open channels, the period during which the bulk of the Na$^+$ is inside and that of the K$^+$ is on the outside is one in which the axon at that point is incapable of being fired. This period of neural incompetence is called the *refractory period*. Within a very short interval, however, the sodium-potassium pump comes back into play, the K$^+$ is again pumped back inside the axon, the Na$^+$ is transported back outside, the membrane is again repolarized in the proper manner, and the axon is again ready to handle another action potential. The period during which the axon cannot accommodate a second action potential, no matter how strong the stimulus, is the *absolute refractory period*. The absolute refractory period is due to the fact that sodium permeability is very low and potassium permeability is quite elevated over normal levels. Immediately following the absolute refractory period as the sodium-potassium pump is again restoring the relative permeabilities of both ions to their original, resting state, the axon may be re-excited by an extra strong stimulus. This period is the *relative refractory period*. However, the action potential in this case is smaller than normal and its propagational velocity is less.

In myelinated fibers, the above process operates only at the nodes of Ranvier, and the nervous impulse is propagated in a saltational manner from node to node. This results in a very rapid movement of the impulse down the axon, since the great majority of the axonal distance "traveled" is *not* through Na$^+$/K$^+$ exchange in the relatively resistant medium of the neural membrane. Rather, the reversal of polarity at one node creates a more or less instantaneous increase in the permeability of the

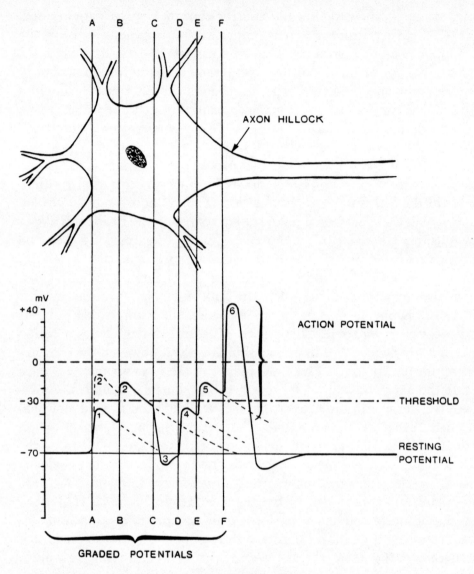

Figure 6
Graded Potentials

Graded potentials vary with the strength and frequency of the stimuli generating them. They are summed algebraically over both time and distance along the soma. When the sum totals of all excitatory and inhibitory potentials reach the axon hillock with an amplitude at or just above the threshold level, an all-or-nothing action potential is generated which sweeps down the axon. The vertical lines A through F represent graded potentials in the graph at the relative points along the lines in the cell body above. Dotted lines represent extinction curves of the potentials had a second potential not been generated which added to the first. 1 = an excitatory potential along line A. 2 = a similar potential along line B — the superposition of 2 above 1 as shown by a dotted curve shows how the two potentials would be summed had they occurred at the same instant. 3=an inhibitory signal and the resulting membrane hyper-polarization is reflected in the inverted spike; its effect is subtractive. 4 and 5 represent two excitatory potentials on lines D and E, respectively. Since the sum of all the potentials exceeds the threshold limit at the axon hillock (F), an action potential (6) is initiated.

---

membrane at the next node down the line, and impulse propagation proceeds by "jumping" from node to node down the length of the axon.

The extracellular region has low electrical resistance as does the *axoplasm* (the cytoplasm within the axon) on the inside of the membrane. The membrane itself, however, is relatively highly resistant to electrical flow, a resistance that is greatly increased by the non-conducting myelin sheath. As Na^+ floods into the axoplasm at one of the nodes of Ranvier, coinciding with the spike of the action potential at that point, the abrupt increase of total internal positive charge causes a massive flow of electrons from the region of the next node "downrange" from the first node. Electrons can flow much more quickly than can the much more massive ions themselves. And the axoplasm is much less resistant to such flow than is the exposed neural membrane to ionic influx or egress. In fact, the axoplasm and external (extracellular) environment function as electrolytes and the flow of electric current from one point to another is for all practical purposes instantaneous.

The sudden stripping away of electrons from the next node of Ranvier along the path of propagation changes the membrane potential of that next region. The loss of electrons results in a net positive charge (that is, a smaller negative charge) inside the membrane because of the now unbalanced positive ionic charges. This polarity reversal causes the sodium gates to open,[6] Na^+ rushes inside, and the events associated with the action potential take place. The action potential thus literally jumps from node to node, completely bypassing the great majority of the length of the myelin-insulated axon. Since the node regions preceding the one at which the action potential is occurring are still in the refractory phase, having already been "fired," they are unable to depolarize and the impulse can therefore proceed in only one direction—namely, from soma to the axonal tip.

In fact, the situation is even more complicated than what I have described. There is a counter-flowing positive current to the negative

---

[6]Sodium and potassium enter and leave the neuron by separate protein channels.

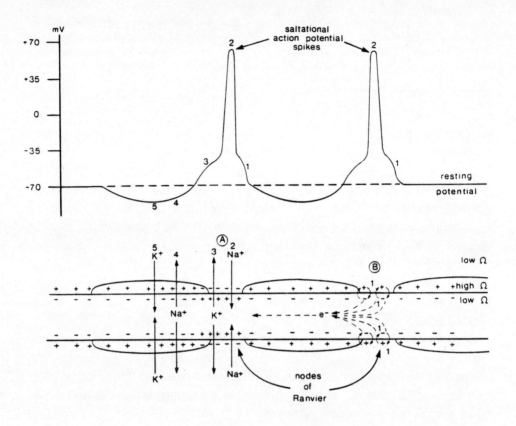

Figure 7
The Action Potential and Saltational
Conduction in Myelinated Fibers

During the action potential, the permeability of the axonal membrane to Na^+ is greatly increased by small electrostatic changes at (1) causing the voltage-gated sodium channels to open. Na^+ floods inside down its concentration gradient causing a sudden reversal in membrane polarity. Within a fraction of a millisecond after they open, the Na^+ gates again close—the resulting action potential spike (2) is due to the period of Na^+ influx. The membrane now becomes extremely permeable to K^+ (3)—even more so than usual—and K^+ flows massively outside down its concentration gradient, re-establishing normal membrane polarity—i.e., positive outside and negative inside; however, the ions are not in their usual respective compartments. During the period between 2 and the establishment of 3, the membrane cannot again be excited; this time of reversed polarity is the absolute refractory period. During period 3, the normal polarity is again established, but because of the excess of K^+ outside the cell relative to the inside, the membrane potential is smaller than normal. This appears as a small trailing hump on the disappearing action potential spike (3) during which subsequent excitation is actually enhanced or facilitated. Very quickly the sodium-potassium pump transports Na^+ back outside and K^+ back inside, thus restoring normal polarity with each of the ions sequestered back into their normal compartments. However, as K^+ are pumped back inside the membrane, they cannot be as rapidly replaced in the extracellular region (especially in the extracellular spaces enclosed by the Schwann cells)—this lag in K^+

replacement (at least up to the normal low concentrations normally present) causes a brief hyperpolarization of the membrane (4 and 5). This period of increased resistance to membrane excitation is the relative refractory period.

The sudden inrushing of Na^+ at point A, resulting in polarity reversal, attracts electrons from ions located further along the path of conduction. Both the extracellular and intracellular media have much lower electrical resistances (here denoted by Ω, for the unit of such resistance, ohm) than does the membrane itself or the enclosing myelin sheath. Both the axoplasm and the interstitial regions thus act as electrolyte solutions, and electron and ion transport there is essentially instantaneous. As the electrons are stripped from their parent ions by the reversed membrane polarity at A and transported from region B to A, a net positive charge results at B since the counterbalancing electrons have been removed. This minor change in electrostatic charge on the inner surface of the membrane at B is sufficient to open the sodium-gates at that point, and a new action potential is generated at node B. The slight depolarization due to the loss of electrons at 1 is represented by the anticipatory hump at the leading edge of the action spike. Action potentials are thus initiated from node to node almost instantaneously, and the nervous impulse is transmitted very rapidly down the length of the axon, effectively bypassing most of it.

Ω = electrical resistance; $\pm$ = region of changing polarity at node B due to Na^+ influx at node A; 1 = slight depolarization causing Na^+ to open; 2 = action potential and opening and closing of Na^+-gates; 3 = K^+ egress; 4 and 5 = resumption of action of Na^+-K^+-pump. Adapted and Modified from Bowman & Rand 1980.

---

current of the electrons, and K^+ ions are believed to flow out into the extracellular medium at the node being perturbed by a depolarizing node more proximal to the soma at the same time that electrons are being stripped away from the perturbed region in the axoplasm. These K^+ may replace calcium ions bound to the *gangliosides* projecting from the membrane into the extracellular environment. The more Ca^{++} there is bound to membrane gangliosides[7] the less permeable the membrane is to other ions. The exchange of some Ca^{++} for K^+ ions causes a conformational change in the membrane channel proteins, allowing Na^+ to flow down its concentration gradient to the inside. At the peak of the action potential, the K^+ bound to the membrane ganliosides are again replaced by Ca^{++}, and the sodium gates slam quickly shut again. This particular portion of the membrane-action potential model is still unclear and is the subject of much controversy and active research efforts. Near their ends axons lose their myelin sheath and give off numerous branches

---

[7]The actual structure of membrane systems is much more complicated than I have described. In addition to the phospholipid bilayer in which are embedded various protein units, a separate protein monolayer covers both surfaces of the membrane, and the outer surface is overlain by a glycoprotein (carbohydrate-protein) coating. Gangliosides are glycolipids (carbohydrate-lipid units) with a negatively charged hydrophilic portion (which binds to cations like K^+ & Ca^{++}) projecting out from the membrane into the extracellular region, and usually a pair of hydrophobic hydrocarbon chains (fatty acids) embedded within the phospholipid bilayer.

which typically are tipped with small button-like knobs or swellings—
the so-called *telodendria* or *terminal buttons* (see figure 1). These terminal
buttons do not actually contact other neurons or other target organs such
as glands or muscle, but are always separated by a very small gap called
the *synapse* in the case of a neuron-neuron junction and which is more
accurately called the *neuro-effector junction* when the "contact" is between
a neuron and another type of tissue or organ. Figure 8 illustrates the
details of the synaptic junction between two neurons.

NEUROTRANSMITTERS AND THE SYNAPSE

The portion of the neuronal membrane at the tip of the terminal
button is referred to as the *presynaptic membrane.* The receiving membrane at the other side of the *synaptic cleft* is called the *postsynaptic
membrane.* Thus far we have been discussing the propagation of a nervous impulse strictly in terms of electrical phenomena. The graded potentials of the soma and the action potential they produce in the axon are
totally electrical in their nature. At the terminal buttons, however, the
incoming electrical potentials precipitate a chain of events which culmi-
nate in the release into the synaptic gap of a chemical agent known as a
neurotransmitter or a *neurotransmitter substance.* Presynaptic (axonal) potentials are *voltage-gated* in that a change in electric potential opens the
channel proteins to their respective ions. Postsynaptic potentials, on the
other hand, are *chemically-gated*—that is specific chemical transmitter
substances diffuse across the synaptic space and combine with highly
specific proteins on the postsynaptic membrane called *receptors.* These
receptors, in turn, may either themselves directly open the sodium and
potassium gates and initiate a nervous impulse in the new neuron (one
messenger system), or they may activate other enzyme systems which
indirectly have that effect (second messenger system).

Chemically-gated potentials have somewhat different properties than
do voltage-gated ones. They are smaller in amplitude, last much longer,
and they are graded according to the amount of neurotransmitter released,
and thus the number of receptors which are activated. One of the most
abundant neurotransmitters is *acetylcholine.* It is synthesized out of choline (one of the vitamins B) and acetyl coenzyme A (see Light 1985)
by the enzyme *choline acetyltransferase.* Both the acetyl coA and the
choline acetyltransferase are synthesized in the cell body of the neuron
and transported to the telodendria by axoplasmic flow. Choline, a polar

cation, does not readily dissolve in the lipid membrane system. It is carried across the membrane of the telodendria from the blood into the terminal button by combining with a carrier protein which transports it into the cell in a process requiring no energy expenditure. Inside the terminal button the acetyl group is removed from acetyl coA by choline acetyltransferase and combined with choline.

Free acetylcholine within the axoplasm of the terminal button is highly vulnerable to attack and hydrolysis by degradation enzymes known as *acetylcholine esterases*. To prevent that the acetylcholine is packaged up into small packets or vesicles in a poorly understood process[8] and stored in the terminal buttons until needed to bridge the synaptic gap. From time to time a vesicle laden with acetylcholine will make random contact with the presynaptic membrane whereupon it fuses with the membrane, and the contents are emptied into the synaptic gap by *exocytosis*. The neurotransmitter thus released bridges the gap and some of the molecules combine with corresponding receptors on the postsynaptic membrane. This causes very small and local postsynaptic depolarizations which, however, are too small to trigger an action potential.

As an action potential sweeps down the axon and enters the terminal button, the change of membrane potential at the button causes voltage-gated Ca^{++} channels to open. The calcium ions are released from their binding sites on the gangliosides, probably by exchange with outflowing K^{+} in a manner like that occurring higher up on the axon. Ca^{++} moves down the concentration gradient and enters the axoplasm of the terminal button. The sudden calcium spike causes a terminal axonal membrane protein, *neurin*, to combine with a similar protein on the vesicular membrane, *stenin*. The vesicular and terminal neuronal membranes thus fuse for a brief period, resulting in the release of the neurotransmitter into the synapse by exocytosis. Precisely similar Ca^{++}—dependent processes are involved in all pinocytotic and secretory or export responses. This causes a very large spike of acetylcholine within the gap because of the large number of vesicles fusing with the presynaptic membrane, and an action potential is generated in the postsynaptic neuron or end organ. As the acetylcholine-laden synaptic vesicles fuse with the presynaptic membrane and release their contents, the Ca^{++} which initiated this

---

[8]The vescicles are presumably made in the cell body and are transported to the terminal buttons by rapid axoplasmic flow involving a protein called *tubulin* which is responsible for cytoplasmic flow in all animal cells.

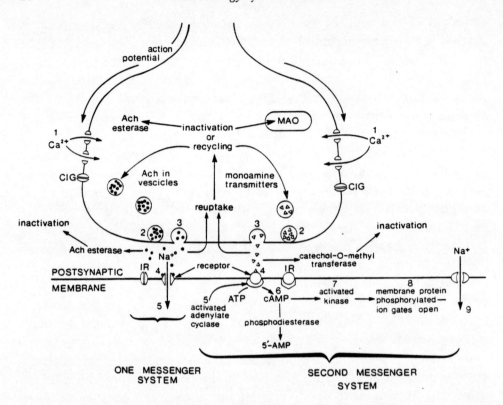

Figure 8
The Synaptic Junction

In the left side of the figure, acetylcholine (Ach) is released into the synaptic cleft, diffuses across to the specific receptor sites, and activates the latter, causing the ionic gates to open. Two acetylcholine molecules are required to open an Ach-mediated gate. Acetylcholine receptors are generally one messenger systems as here illustrated; in the limbic system, cholinergic receptors are typically second messenger systems (primarily involving guanylate cyclase and cyclic guanosine monophosphate). GABA also usually operates on a one messenger basis. The right side of the figure represents the two messenger system involved in all of the monoamine and oligopeptide neurotransmitter-receptor interactions. The receptor is coupled to adenylate cyclase which, when activated, transforms ATP into cAMP. The cAMP then activates a protein kinase, which phosphorylates a membrane protein causing its ionic gate moiety to open. Although Na^+ is shown as the cation entering the postsynaptic channel, other inorganic ions, especially Cl^-, may also be involved, particularly at inhibitory synapses.

(1) calcium gates in terminal button open in response to action potential; (2) Ca^{2+} spike causes synaptic vesicles to fuse with presynaptic membrane of terminal button; (3) exocytosis and release of neurotransmitter into synaptic cleft; (4) binding of neurotransmitter to specific receptor—acetylcholine and single messenger system shown on left, and the two messenger system activated by the monoamine and oligopeptide neurotransmitters is depicted on the right; (5 et seq.) the event or chain of events initiated by the binding of neurotransmitter to the receptor—on the left, receptor activation directly opens specific ion channels, on the right, the attached enzyme, adenylate cyclase is activated, which in turn converts ATP into cAMP; (7) protein kinase is activated by cAMP; (8) activated protein kinase phosphorylates membrane

protein, causing ion channel to open (9); π = unactivated ion channels or postsynaptic receptors.

Once synaptic transmission has been effected, the transmitter substances are broken down or reabsorbed by the presynaptic terminal to prevent uncontrolled firing of the postsynaptic fiber. Acetylcholine is broken down into its acetyl and choline moieties by acetylcholine esterase which is present both in the synaptic cleft and the axoplasm of the presynaptic terminal. The monoamine neurotransmitters (dopamine, norepinephrine, and serotonin) are destroyed by catechol-O-methyltransferase within the synaptic cleft; that which is reabsorbed by the presynaptic terminal is either recycled back into protective vesicles for re-use, or destroyed within the terminal mitochondria by monoamine oxidase. In the absence of adenylate cyclase activation, cAMP is spontaneously inactivated by the enzyme cyclic nucleotide phosphodiesterase. Adapted and modified from Iversen 1979.

---

process are rapidly sequestered and actively exported out of the terminal button to the extracellular region where they again bind loosely with the gangliosides in exchange for the K^+, which are now pumped back into the axoplasm by the sodium-potassium pump.

As the acetylcholine spike activates the receptors on the postsynaptic membrane, it is almost immediately deactivated by the enzyme acetylcholinesterase. This prevents the postsynaptic membrane from firing repeatedly due to the continued presence of the neurotransmitter in the synaptic cleft. Such repeated, uncontrolled firing would lead to seizures in very short order. Once released into the synapse the acetylcholine is no longer protected by the membranes of the synaptic vesicles, and it is very quickly degraded. The acetylcholinesterase strips the acetyl group ($CH_3-\underset{O}{C}-$) from the choline moiety in a hydrolytic reaction (one which absorbs water), producing choline and acetic acid (figure 9A). Acetylcholinesterase can cleave 25,000 molecules of acetylcholine per second (Iversen 1979).

Each synaptic vesicle contains about 10,000 molecules of acetylcholine and these molecules bind to the acetylcholine receptor sites on the postsynaptic membrane within 100 microseconds (0.0001 second) (Stevens 1979). There is always a great deal more neurotransmitter released into the synaptic cleft than there are acetylcholine receptors. It requires two acetylcholine molecules to activate one postsynaptic receptor, and each presynaptic vesicle of 10,000 acetylcholine molecules can activate about 2,000 postsynaptic receptors (Stevens 1979). When two acetylcholine molecules bind to a given receptor site, that protein undergoes a change in stereochemical conformation due to a lowered energy state resulting from the binding of the neurotransmitter. The acetylcholine receptor bears ion-channels specific for Na^+ and K^+. The activated receptor suddenly opens its channels, the Na^+ flood in and the K^+ pour out through the postsynaptic membrane and the resulting depolarization of the membrane triggers a graded potential. Once the acetylcholine is dissociated from the receptor, the Na^+ channel closes and the resting potential is quickly restored by the sodium-potassium pump. These graded potentials vary in both amplitude and frequency depending upon the amount at acetylcholine released into the synapse. The number of synaptic vesicles released by the presynaptic membrane in turn depends upon the number of action potentials per unit time which enter the terminal button.[9] The number of postsynaptic receptors activated also depend upon the number of axons impinging upon the soma and dendrites of the neuron in question.[10]

There are three other major neurotransmitter substances in the CNS known as *monoamines*—substances synthesized from specific amino acids within the terminal buttons of the neurons which secrete them. The monoamines are so named because of the single amine ($-NH_2$) group carried by the amino acid precursors and their derivatives. Additionally, a number of short peptide chains called *oligopeptides* (protein fragments) which have a variety of functions as hormones in the body also play important roles as neurotransmitters in the brain (more about this below).[11]

Dopamine and *norepinephrine* (*noradrenalin*) are both synthesized from the same amino acid precursor, *tyrosine*. The amino acid and its two neurotransmitter derivatives have the same basic structure—a benzene ring (phenyl group) attached to a two-carbon (ethyl group) chain bearing an amine group. This class of structures is known as a *beta-phenylethylamine* (see figure 9B). Dopamine and norepinephrine are both *catecholamines*. These neurotransmitters tend to be excitatory, that is they generate an excitatory postsynaptic potential; however they also have an inhibitory effect under some circumstances. Tyrosine, like choline, is transported across the membrane of the terminal button by a carrier protein. Once inside the axoplasm it is acted upon by specific enzymes produced in the cell body and transported down to the terminal button by axoplasmic

---

[9]It will be recalled that the number of all-or-nothing action potentials generated per unit time is a direct function of the strength of the initiating stimulus.

[10]A given neuron may have 1,000–10,000 synapses and be innervated by about 1,000 other neurons (Stevens 1979).

[11]Hormones are substances secreted by specific tissues or cells which are carried by the blood and which affect specific target tissues or cells at a distance from the point of origin of the substance.

flow.[12] Tyrosine (figure 9B) is converted by tyrosine hydroxylase into the compound *L–DOPA* or *levodopa*. In this process a specific phenyl hydrogen atom is removed and replaced by an −OH group. L–DOPA is then converted by *dopa decarboxylase* into the neurotransmitter dopamine in a reaction in which the carboxyl group (−COOH) is removed and a hydrogen atom is added. Dopamine is a powerful neurotransmitter itself, and it plays many important roles in the brain in that capacity. Dopamine is in turn transformed into norepinephrine by the enzyme *dopamine-beta-hydroxylase*. In this process, one of the hydrogen atoms on the beta-carbon atom of the ethylamine side chain is replaced by a hydroxyl group. The relative levels of norepinephrine relative to dopamine are very important in the etiology of several major emotional disorders as well as neurological motor disturbances. Disulfiram (Antabuse®) inhibits the activity of dopamine-beta-hydroxylase, thus lowering the levels of norepinephrine and contributing to the disulfiram-ethanol toxic reaction (see Light 1985).

In a very similar manner, the neurotransmitter *serotonin* or *5-hydroxytryptamine (5-HT)* is synthesized in two steps from the amino acid precursor, *tryptophan*. Unlike dopamine and norepinephrine, serotonin is a complex ring structure consisting of a phenyl group, an attached 5-sided, nitrogen-bearing ring, plus an attached alkyl group (hydrocarbon chain) with a terminal amine group (figure 9C). Such a structure is called an *indole* or *indolealkylamine*, and unlike the beta-phenylethylamines dopamine and norepinephrine, has primarily an inhibitory effect upon CNS neurons. Together with norepinephrine, as we shall see presently, it regulates waking, sleep, and dreaming activity and both are involved in the etiology of primary depressive disorder. The transformation of tryptophan into serotonin or 5-HT is exactly analogous to the production of dopamine from tyrosine. The tryptophan is first hydroxylated by *tryptophan-5-hydroxylase* into the intermediate compound, *5-hydroxytryptophan* (also known as *5-hydroxyindoleacetate* or *5-HIAA*). This intermediate is then decarboxylated by *5-hydroxytryptophan decarboxylase* into 5-hydroxytryptamine or serotonin.

The monoamine neurotransmitters, and acetylcholine, are packaged

[12]Keep in mind that enzymes, being proteins, can only be synthesized by mRNA together with tRNA and their associated amino acids on ribosomes. These ribosomes are found only in the somae of nerve cells. However, the monoamines themselves are readily synthesized within the terminal buttons out of their precursor amino acids in a series of two or three steps catalyzed by the enzymes produced in the somae and carried to the terminals.

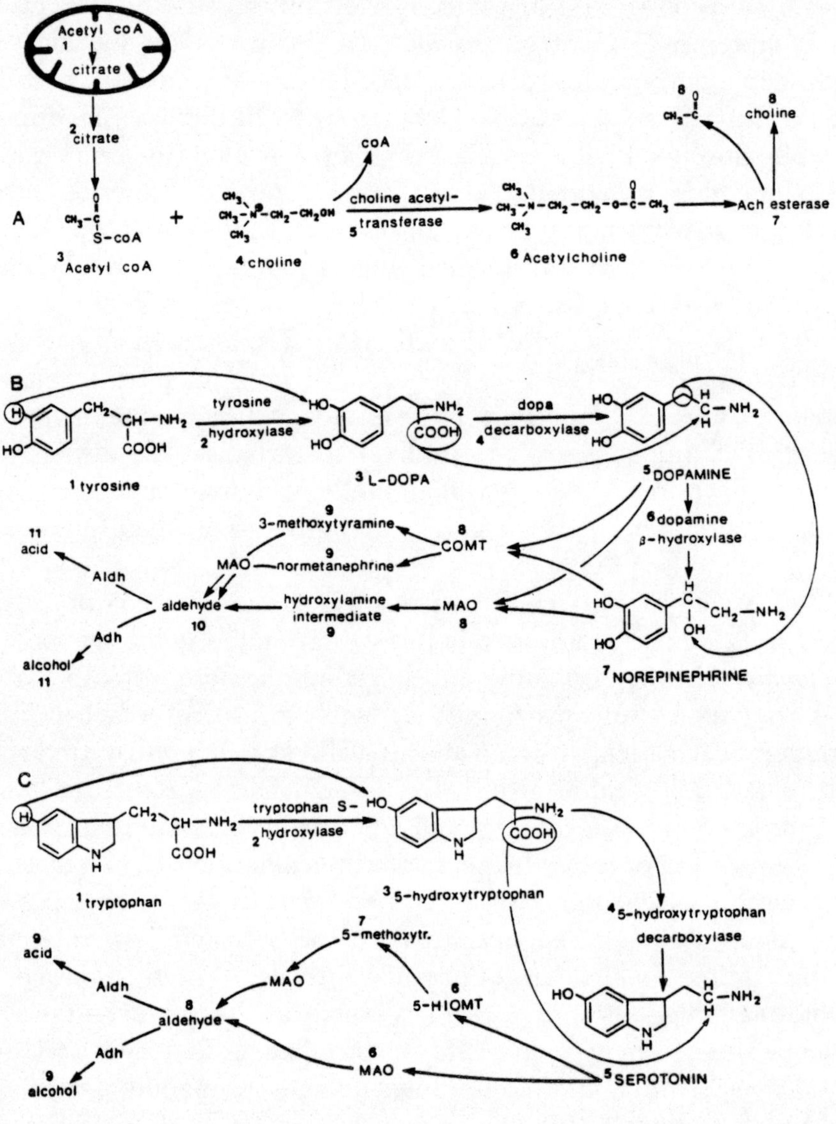

Figure 9
Acetylcholine and Monoamine Synthesis and Catabolism

The synthesis of acetylcholine, the β-phenylethylamines dopamine and norepinephrine, and the indole-alkylamine serotonin takes place within the presynaptic terminal button. The precursor amino acids are taken up from the blood by carrier proteins and transported inside the axon terminal. The enzymes facilitating the various synthesis and degradative processes are synthesized along ribosomes within the cell body and transported to the terminal by axoplasmic flow.

A. Acetyl co-A cannot be transported across the mitochondrial membrane. Therefore in order to be available for the synthesis of acteylcholine, it is first converted into citrate

(1), carried across the mitochondrial wall (2) and then re-converted back into acetyl co-A via the exact same steps involved in lipogenesis (see Light 1985, for discussion). Acetyl coA (3) combines with a vitamin, choline, (4) in the presence of choline acetyltransferase (5), releasing a free co-A and forming acteylcholine (6). Acetylcholine, in turn, is degraded by acetylcholine esterase (7) into the original constituents (8).

B. β-phenylethylamine synthesis from the amino acid tyrosine. Tyrosine (1) is hydroxylated at the number 3-carbon by tyrosine hydroxylase (2) to form L–DOPA (3). The carboxyl group is removed from L–DOPA by dopa decarboxylase (4) to form the potent neurotransmitter dopamine (5). The enzyme dopamine-β-hydroxylase (6) is not present in dopaminergic neurons and this process stops here. The enzyme is, however, present in norepinephrine-containing neurons bound to the membranes of the storage vesicles. In such neurons dopamine is hydroxylated into norepinephrine (7) and stored within the presynaptic vesicles until needed for synaptic transmission. Both dopamine and norepinephrine are degraded by monoamine oxidase (MAO) and catechol-O-methyltransferase (COMT) into their respective aldehydes (8–10). In turn the aldehyde is either oxidized into its respective acid or reduced into its alcohol (11) (see also figures 25 and 26). The presence of large amounts of ethanol and its metabolite acetaldehyde can seriously disrupt this degradative process and stimulate the production of powerful neurotropic condensation products, the tetrahydroisoquinolines. C. Serotonin (5-hydroxytryptamine or 5-HT) synthesis. In a process very much like the above, the amino acid tryptophan (1) is hydroxylated by tryptophan-S-hydroxylase (2) into 5-hydroxytryptophan (3) [= 5-hydroxyindoleacetate 5-HIAA], which in turn is converted into serotonin by decarboxylation (4 and 5). Serotonin is degraded by MAO and 5-hydroxyindole-O-methyltransferase [5-HIOMT] (6 and 7) into 5-hydroxyindole-3-acetaldehyde (8) which is then converted into its acid (5-HIAA) and its alcohol [5-hydroxytryptophol or 5-HTOL] (9). The condensation products deriving from ethanol challenge are tetrahydro-beta-carbolines. MAO = monoamine oxidase; COMT = catechol-O-methyltransferase; 5-HIOMT = 5-hydroxyindole-O-methyltransferase; Ald = aldehyde dehydrogenase; Adh = alcohol dehydrogenase. The large arrowheads indicate biosynthetic or degradative pathways. The small arrowheads indicate the site upon the precursor molecule and the product at which the enzyme acts in each case.

---

up inside synaptic vesicles to prevent their breakdown by inactivating enzymes, and they are similarly released into the synaptic cleft by the action of inflowing Ca^{++} in response to a presynaptic action potential. They each bind to highly specific postsynaptic receptor sites. Unlike acetylcholine, however, they are inactivated only partially within the synaptic cleft after binding to the receptors. Most monoamine neurotransmitters are resorbed back into the presynaptic terminal button by *endocytosis*, the exact reverse process to exocytosis. Once back inside the terminal button, the monoamines are degraded by the enzymes *monoamine oxidase* or *MAO* and *catechol-O-methyltransferase* (or *5-hydroxyindole-O-methyltransferase* in the case of serotonin). MAO operates primarily within the mitochondria contained in the axoplasm of the terminal button. Catechol-O-methyltransferase (COMT) operates both within the synaptic cleft and the axoplasm of the terminal button. A significant portion of the resorbed monoamine neurotransmitter is also usually repackaged within synaptic vesicles and stored for subsequent re-use (figure 8).

Whereas acetylcholine constitutes a primary messenger which opens the post-synaptic sodium-potassium gates directly, all the monoamines operate primarily by way of a *second messenger system* to either open or close the ionic gates specific to the receptors being acted upon (figure 8). The monoamine receptor site is closely attached to a specific enzyme, *adenylate cyclase,* which converts ATP into cyclic AMP. The cAMP in turn activates a protein kinase[13] and this activated kinase causes the phosphorylation (and thus the activation) of the target protein. During periods when the receptors involved in this second messenger system are not activated, cAMP is quickly inactivated by *cyclic nucleotide phosphodiesterase* which converts cAMP into non-cyclic *5'-AMP* (see figure 8).[14]

There are thus two basic types of neurotransmitter receptors: (1) rapid acting receptors which directly control the permeability of their respective ion-pores, and (2) longer acting receptors which activate a second messenger (usually adenylate cyclase) which in turn mediates the effect of the neurotransmitter inside the target neuron in a complex manner. Transmitter substances may have more than one type of receptor. An example is acetylcholine. In the peripheral nervous system, for example at the junction between a motor neuron and a muscle endplate, the sodium gates are directly opened when the acetylcholine receptors are bound by the neurotransmitter. The amino acid GABA (see below) also operates in this way. As suggested in footnote[13], however, cholinergic neurons within the brain itself are depolarized via another second messenger system, this time involving guanylate cyclase which converts the closely related nucleotide phosphate, *guanosine triphosphate (GTP)* into *cyclic guanosine monophosphate (cGMP).* The effects of *cGMP* upon protein kinases are exactly equivalent to the action of cAMP. Furthermore, dopamine also acts upon two types of receptors in the brain: (1) D_2 *receptors,* which directly mediate membrane permeability and Na^+ influx,

---

[13]Adenylate cyclase and cAMP are the second messengers in nearly all cell processes throughout the body. Cyclic AMP activates a wide variety of protein kinases, each of which affects a specific, membrane-bound protein. This system is involved in all alterations of membrane permeability, mechanical effects, synthesis, secretion, glycogenolysis, and lipolysis. A very similar system involving *guanylate cyclase, guanosine triphosphate* and *cGMP* operates in acetylcholinergic neurons within the brain itself.

[14]See also below, figure 24 and associated text.

and (2) D_1 *receptors*, which are coupled to the second messenger cAMP system (by far the most abundant type of dopamine receptors).

Two major types of postsynaptic potentials are generated by the diffusion of neurotransmitters across the synaptic cleft resulting in the activation of specific receptor sites (figure 10):

(1) **Excitatory Postsynaptic Potentials (EPSP)** are produced when the activated neurotransmitter receptor causes a *depolarization* of the postsynaptic membrane. Generalized ionic gates open in response to receptor activation which permit the influx of Na^+ from outside the cell membrane and efflux of K^+ to the exterior. The net result is membrane depolarization (not reversal, as in the case of an axonal action potential) as Na^+ and K^+ rush through the now permeable membrane down their respective concentration gradients. This depolarization produces an excitatory graded potential in the postsynaptic medium which can be summed in the usual way, and which leads to an action potential when present in sufficient combined strength.

(2) **Inhibitory Postsynaptic Potentials (IPSP)** occur when the activation of receptors by the neurotransmitter causes a *hyperpolarization* of the postsynaptic membrane. This is accomplished by an increased *selective* permeability of the membrane allowing K^+ efflux and Cl^- influx via specific channels. The increased minus charge on the inside due to inflowing Cl^- relative to the enhanced positive charge outside resulting from K^+ egress renders the membrane much less likely to respond to stimulation by excitatory receptors with depolarization and the generation of a graded potential.

Both inhibitory and excitatory nerve terminals impinge upon the dendrites and cell bodies of most neurons, each with their respective neurotransmitters and specific postsynaptic receptor sites. It will be recalled that the total number of excitatory and inhibitory postsynaptic responses are algebraically summed over both distance and time (figure 6), which determines the net effect at the axon hillock.

In addition to acetylcholine and the monoamines dopamine, norepinephrine and serotonin, a number of amino acids and peptide sequences serve as important CNS neurotransmitters. Among the amino acids, *glutamic acid* or *glutamate* and *aspartic acid* or *aspartate* exert a strong excitatory effect upon most CNS neurons. Conversely, *glycine* and *gamma-aminobutyric acid* or *GABA* (derived from glutamate) are powerful inhibitory neurotransmitters in the brain. In fact, GABA is the commonest inhibitory substance in the brain, being used as a transmitter in nearly one-third of

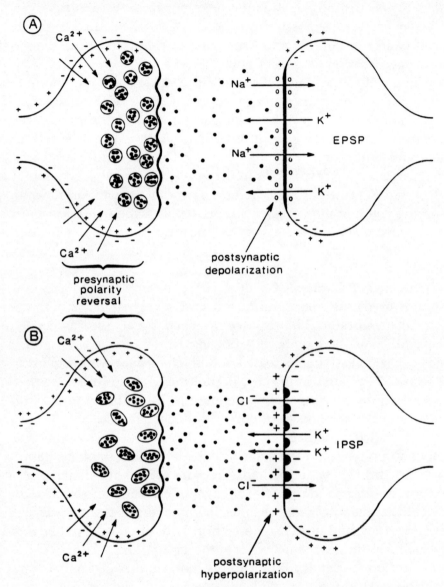

Figure 10
Excitatory and Inhibitory Postsynaptic Potentials

The action potential causes a reversal in membrane polarity as it moves into the presynaptic terminal, thus opening ionic gates and allowing Ca^{2+} to enter the terminal, releasing neurotransmitter into the synaptic cleft.

A. Generalized ionic gates are opened allowing Na^+ and K^+ to flow inward and outward, respectively, down their concentration gradients, depolarizing the postsynaptic membrane and generating an excitatory postsynaptic potential (EPSP). B. Only very selective ionic gates are opened, K$^+$ flow outside and Cl$^-$ flow inward down their respective concentration gradients which augments the net negative charge inside relative to the positive charge outside. This membrane hyperpolarization generates an inhibitory postsynaptic potential (IPSP).

---

all brain synapses, and it is unique among amino acids in being synthesized almost entirely within the brain and spinal cord.[15]

A number of peptide sequences which serve as important hormones within the body also function as specific neurotransmitters in the brain. Neurons secreting these oligopeptides are called *peptidergic* neurons. *Substance P* causes contraction of smooth muscle within the gastrointestinal tract and it stimulates peristaltic movements of the intestine. It has a vasodilational effect upon vascular smooth muscle and causes a drop in blood pressure. It is widely distributed in the small intestine, brain and spinal cord. In neural tissue it mediates the perception of pain (figure 11), particularly in association with neurons in the dorsal root ganglia (see below), the spinal tracts, and the thalamus, hippocampus, substantia nigra, hypothalamus, and selected cortical parts of the brain. The body's endogenous opiate-like agents appear to act by suppressing the secretion of substance P (see below). Other putative (suspected) peptide neurotransmitters with other hormonal functions outside the nervous system include:

angiotensin II—the most powerful vasoconstrictor and hypertensive agent in the body; when injected into the brain it percipitates intense and prolonged drinking behavior despite adequate body hydration.

cholecystokinin (CCK) [=*pancreozymin (PZ)*]—as a hormone CCK works together with secretin (see Light 1985) to initiate secretion of pancreatic juice, and is itself stimulated by secretin; it also exists in the hypothalamus where it probably acts as a neurotransmitter substance.

vasoactive intestinal peptide—related to glucagon and secretin; it is also found in the frontal lobe cerebral cortex and in the hypothalamus.

somatostatin (growth hormone release-inhibiting hormone)—released by the hypothalamus to regulate hormone secretion by the anterior lobe of the pituitary gland (see below), it inhibits the release of growth hormone (somatotropin), prolactin, follicle stimulating hormone, and

---

[15]A specific deficit of GABA is responsible for Huntington's chorea, a genetically inherited, progressive and nearly always fatal disease characterized by involuntary, but coordinated movements, mental deterioration and severe psychosis.

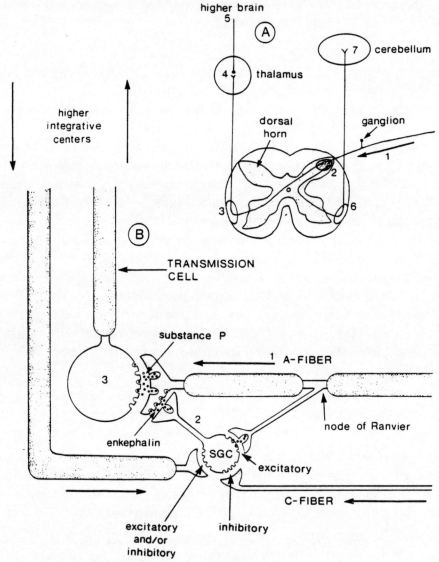

Figure 11
Enkephalin and Substance P Axo-axonal Interaction

A. A pain stimulus is conducted to the CNS along a primary sensory neuron (1) and enters the substantia gelatinosa (2) located within the dorsal horns of the spinal gray matter (lightly stippled "X"). The primary sensory neuron forms synapses within the substantia gelatinosa and the impulse is transmitted to the higher portions of the CNS via several spinal routes: the impulse travels to the thalamic "relay station" (4) via the lateral spinothalamic tract (3) on the opposite side of the spinal cord from the incoming pain signal. The thalamus then forwards the signal to the appropriate portions of the cerebral cortex (5) for perception, integration and processing; the signal is also sent via the anterior spinocerebellar tract (6) on the same side as the incoming impulse to the cerebellum (7). B. Expanded detail of A. Sharp, intense pain signals are rapidly conducted to the substantia gelatinosa via myelinated A-fibers (1). The A-fiber releases substance P at its synapse with the secondary spinal, pain-receiving neuron or transmission cell (3) for conduction to the higher integrative brain centers. An enkephalin-releasing substantia gelatinosa cell (SGC) makes axo-axonal "contact" with the terminus of the A-fiber (2), and it is itself innervated by a collateral branch of the A-fiber's axon. When stimulated by the collateral branch of the A-fiber, the SGC releases enkephalin which is taken up by the mu-receptors on the A-fiber's terminal button. This inhibits the secretion of substance P by the A-fiber and decreases the transmission of the pain impulse to the higher brain centers by the transmission cell. The A-fiber-SGC-transmission cell complex thus comprises a negative feedback system by which pain impulses from the A-fiber modulate their own intensity of subsequent spinal transmission. Non-myelinated C-fibers carry slower, more diffuse, aching, "duller" pain signals. They also activate the transmission cell (not figured here) and exert an inhibitory effect upon the SGC. Signals from the brain convey excitatory and/or inhibitory effects upon the SGC. Similar interactions occur in both the mu- and delta-receptors in the limbic system of the brain which is concerned with the perception and regulation of emotions. Adapted from several drawings in Iversen 1979 and Bowman & Rand 1980.

---

thyrotropin (thyroid stimulating hormone), as well as insulin and glucagon from the pancreas and gastrin from the stomach; somatostatin has been found in many areas of the cerebral cortex where it has been specifically identified as associated with synapses.

thyrotropin release-inhibiting hormone (TR-IH) or *thyroptropin regulating hormone (TRH)*—secreted by the hypothalamus to regulate the anterior pituitary, this peptide is widespread in the CNS where it potentiates the action of acetylcholine; it is antagonistic to the action of barbiturates (White et al 1978).

By far the most important of the oligopeptide neurotransmitters with respect to the action of psychotropic drugs are the *enkephalins* and *endorphins,* endogenous "opioids" which bind to the same receptor sites which accept artificially introduced opiates such as morphine, heroin and codeine. In fact, it was the presence of specific receptor sites in the CNS for these narcotic agents that led to the discovery of the enkephalins and endorphins.[16] The first of these to be discovered were two pentapeptides (peptides five amino acids long) which differed from each other

---

[16]The very fact that such highly specific receptors for narcotic drugs existed in the human CNS implied the existence of endogenous substances which must bind to these same receptors and produce the same effects (analgesia, euphoria, and emotional tranquility). The discovery of morphine receptors in the early 1970's launched a large-scale search for the endogenous "opioids" that had to exist to interact with these receptors. The search was quickly rewarded and led to the current model by which analgesia is produced by such agents, as well as by the naturally occurring endorphins.

only by one of the terminal amino acids. *Met-enkephalin* (*methionine-enkephalin*) has the sequence: tyrosine- glycine-glycine-phenylalanine-methionine. *Leu-enkephalin* (*leucine-enkephalin*) has the sequence: tyrosine-glycine-glycine-phenylalanine-leucine. Met-enkephalin binds to the so-called *mu-receptors* which are abundantly distributed in the layers of the cerebral cortex involved in integrating sensory perception, the thalamus (see below), and the hippocampus. There are also many mu-receptors in the *substantia gelatinosa* (figure 11A) of the spinal cord. These receptors mediate analgesia and they are the same receptors which bind to narcotic drugs. *Delta-receptors* are widely distributed in the nucleus accumbens, olfactory tubercles and amygdala of the *limbic system*[17] which is involved in the regulation of the emotions. Delta-receptors bind with leu-enkephalins and help to mediate emotional tranquility and euphoria. The caudate nucleus (one of the basal ganglia of the limbic system) and the substantia gelatinosa of the spinal cord contain equal distributions of met- and leu-enkephalins and of the mu- and delta-receptors which respectively bind to them.

The endogenous enkephalins appear to act by inhibiting the release of substance P and other neurotransmitters such as acetylcholine at specific synapses along the spinal and cranial pathways involved in the perception and experience of pain and dysphoria (unpleasant emotional experiences). Enkephalin-secreting neurons make axo-axonal synapses with substance-P secreting, pain-mediating neurons (figure 11B). The transmission of pain is produced by the pre-synaptic release of substance P in response to an action potential generated in a pain fiber by a peripheral receptor. When enkephalins are released into the axoaxonal synaptic gap, they bind to specific receptor sites on the postsynaptic axon terminal and prevent the release of substance P by that pain-transmitting neuron. This diminishes or blocks altogether the propagation of painful or unpleasant stimuli farther along the pathway of transmission than that point. Exogenous opiates such as heroin, morphine and codeine also bind to and activate these same receptors and mimic the action of the enkephalins. Both the endogenous enkephalins and the exogenous opiates appear to act upon substance P releasing neurons by altering Na^+ permeability and/or by diminishing the activity of adenylate cyclase.

----

[17]The limbic system is an association of structures derived from the paleocortex or "old cerebral cortex"; it underlies the neocortex ("new cortex") and envelopes the lower forebrain, midbrain and hindbrain structures such as the thalamus, hypothalamus, reticular formation, etc. These structures and their functions are treated later in this section.

There are several important differences in the way in which acetylcholine, the catecholamines and serotonin are synthesized and operate relative to the several peptide transmitters. The amino acid based transmitters and acetylcholine are synthesized in two or three simple steps within the axon terminals by enzymes which are themselves created in the cell bodies and which are transported to the terminals by axoplasmic flow. This class of neurotransmitters acts by altering postsynaptic membrane permeability to ions; they are either excitatory or inhibitory and either decrease or increase voltage gradients, respectively. In contrast the synthesis of peptide transmitters is extremely complex. It can occur only within the cell bodies of neurons and it requires the transcription of mRNA from nuclear DNA and involves tRNA and the stepwise building up of a sequence of peptide bonds by ribosomes (see footnote[1], and Light in press, Volume 4). The peptides must then be carried to the axon terminals by axoplasmic flow before they can be utilized in neural transmission. Peptide transmitters are first synthesized as parts of much larger protein chains. They are then selectively cleaved by specific enzymes into their functional subunits.[18] Peptide messengers act by making the target cells less likely to respond to other signals: (1) they can keep excitatory transmitters from depolarizing the postsynaptic membrane, and (2) can keep inhibitory transmitters from hyperpolarizing the postsynaptic membrane. They thus act by *disenabling* the postsynaptic membrane's competence to respond to other signals.

THE PITUITARY

A final class of neurotransmission occurs in the so-called *neuroendocrine transducers* (figure 12A). These neurons terminate in bulbous axonal endings rather than the terminal buttons typical of most nerve cells. These bulbous terminals contain both neurotransmitter vesicles and *neurosecretory vesicles;* the latter contain special neurohormones which are released into the blood for action on target tissues at a distance from the site of release. The bulbous terminals lie close alongside and actually

---

[18]For example, the pentapeptide enkephalins are part of the longer, 33-amino acid *beta-endorphin*, which in turn forms a small part of the much longer *beta-lipotropin*. In turn, beta-lipotropin together with *corticotropin* and *gamma-melanocyte stimulating hormone* (γ-MSH) and several other amino acid sequences make up the very long precursor protein, *pro-opiomelanocortin*. Endorphins occur in neurons in the base of the hypothalamus and in the anterior pituitary where they exert enkephalinlike actions. Lipotropin is a hormone involved in fat catabolism, and MSH promotes the secretion of GABA and serotonin in the mid-brain and hypothalamus.

contact the capillaries; this neurocapillary complex is known as a *neurohaemal organ*. As an action potential sweeps into the neurohaemal terminal of such a neuron, calcium ions are caused to flow into the terminal in the usual way and they initiate the release of one or another neurotransmitter *within the axonal bulb itself* from the storage vesicles. The release of transmitter molecules acts upon the neurosecretory vesicles also residing within the axonal bulb, and causes the latter to release their specific neurohormones into the blood stream.

Such neuroendocrine transducers occur in great abundance in the hypothalamus where they secrete neurohormones that act specifically upon the anterior lobe of the pituitary gland or upon cells and tissues elsewhere in the body. The hypothalamus comprises the floor of the lower forebrain (figure 16), whose sidewalls are formed by the left and right thalamus. Near its center the hypothalamus projects downward in a deep outpocketing or vertical evagination (figures 12B and 16) known as the *infundibulum*. The anterior or forward wall of the infundibulum bears a prominent swelling, the *median eminence*, beneath which lies the anterior and middle lobes of the pituitary gland—the *adenohypophysis* (*pars distalis*) and the *pars intermedia*, respectively. Lying above and forward of the median eminence is the large tract of fibers where the nerves from the right and left eyeballs cross over to the opposite sides of the brain—the *optic chiasma*. The *anterior hypophyseal artery* enters the median eminence of the hypothalamus where it forms a series of loops called the *primary plexus*. From the primary plexus vessels run down from the median eminence and into the adenohypophysis where they drain into a large capillary network and which ultimately opens into the general circulation again. This vascular complex is called the *hypothalamic-hypophyseal portal system*, and like all portal systems (for example, see Light 1985 with regard to the hepatic portal system), it functions as a direct route of transportation of substances from the median eminence into the adenohypophysis—specifically for neurohormones secreted by hypothalamic neuroendocrine transducers which are directed at the adenohypophysis. Monoamine secreting neurons impinge from elsewhere in the brain upon such neuroendocrine neurons concentrated within the *arcuate* and *tuberal nuclei* within the median eminence. These monoamine releasing neurons cause the neuroendocrine transducers to release their hormones directly into the hypothalamic-hypophyseal portal system through the neurohaemal organs. The neurohormones are transported directly to the anterior pituitary where they cause special endocrine cells to secrete their products into the capillary plexus for transport out of the pituitary and into the general circulation for action at distant target tissues. Drugs which alter the effects of monoamine neurotransmitters, for example chlorpromazine (Thorazine®) which blocks the effects of dopamine, may operate in the nuclei of the median eminence and cause pituitary dysfunction, resulting, for example, in failure to ovulate.

The posterior or rear wall of the infundibulum forms the *posterior lobe* of the pituitary, also known as the *neurohypophysis* or *pars nervosa.*[19] A similar but much smaller portal complex enters and leaves the neurohypophysis near the apex. Neuroendocrine transducers run from the *supraoptic nuclei* located just above and behind the optic chiasma, as well as from the *paraventricular nuclei* located just above the mammillary bodies (see figure 12B, 19 and text below). These transducer neurons secrete *vasopressin* or *antidiuretic hormone* and *oxytocin* into this vascular complex for transportation to (1) the kidneys and (2) the mammary glands and uterus, respectively, where both act. Several of the peptide hormone/neurotransmitter substances listed on pages 29 and 31 are released from the hypothalamus via these two mechanisms.

Those hormones which are released from the median eminence into the hypothalamic-hypophyseal portal system for action in the adenophyophysis are called *hypophysiotropic hormones.* They stimulate the anterior pituitary to release such important hormones as: thyroid-stimulating hormone (TSH) which activates the thyroid gland to produce thyroxine; growth hormone (somatotropin) which stimulates the growth of skeletal and muscular structures, initiates puberty and promotes the onset of REM-sleep (see below); adrenocorticotropic hormone (ACTH) or corticotropin which causes the adrenal cortex to release steroids in response to stress; and gonadotropic hormones such as follicle stimulating hormone (FSH) which causes follicle maturation and ovulation in females and testosterone synthesis in males, and luteinizing hormone (LH) which maintains the corpus luteum and progesterone output in females and

[19]The adenohypophysis is derived from an outpocket of the roof of the embryonic mouth known as *Rathke's pouch.* This pocket eventually separates from the palate and migrates to the hypothalamus where it fuses to form the anterior pituitary lobe. The middle lobe derives from the lower anterior wall of the infundibulum and that wall of Rathke's pouch that fuses with it. The adenohypophysis is thus formed out of embryonic buccal ectoderm whereas the pars intermedia arises jointly from buccal ectoderm and neural ectoderm from the floor of the brain (hypothalamus). The posterior pituitary arises entirely from the hypothalamus; because it consists entirely of neural ectoderm it is called the neurohypophysis or pars nervosa. See also Light (in press, Volume 4).

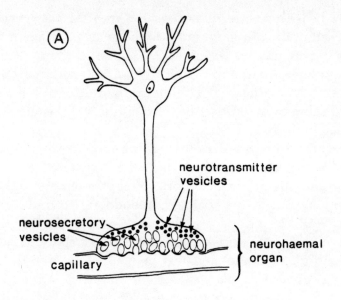

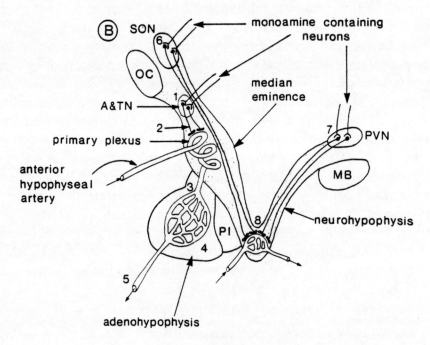

Figure 12
Pituitary Portal System

A. Neuroendocrine transducer cell showing bulbous axonal ending in direct contact with
capillary, forming a neurohaemal organ. An action potential triggers the release of neuro-

transmitter from the storage vesicles, which in turn causes the neurosecretory vesicles to release their neurohormone into the blood. B. Hypthalamic-hypophyseal portal system. Monoamine secreting neurons synapse with neuroendocrine transducers whose somae are located in the arcuate and tuberal nuclei (1), causing the latter to release their hypophysiotropic hormones (release-stimulating or release-inhibiting factors) into the hypophyseal portal system (2). These hypophysiotropic hormones are carried by the portal system into the adenohypophysis or anterior pituitary (3), where they stimulate or inhibit the release of hormones by endocrine secretory cells (4). These hormones are then carried into the rest of the body (5) for action at specific targets at a distance. The posterior pituitary or neurohypophysis contains an analogous system. Incoming signals cause neuroendocrine transducers whose somae are located in the supraoptic (6) and paraventricular (7) nuclei to release oxytocin and vasopressin, respectively, into the blood (8) for action at distant target tissues or organs. A&TN = arcuate and tuberal nuclei; SON = supraoptic nuclei; PVN = paraventricular nuclei; OC = optic chiasma; MB = mamillary bodies; PI = pars intermedia or middle lobe of the pituitary.

---

which is necessary to the maturation of spermatozoa in males. These hypophysiotropic hormones interact with the pituitary and secondary target organs in a *cascading amplifier system* whereby minute amounts of monoamine neurotransmitters in the hypothalamus initiate the secretion of many more molecules of releasing factors or hypophysiotropins which are carried to the adenohypophysis. There they cause the release of a thousand to a million times as much organotropic hormone which in turn stimulates the target organs to produce yet another thousand or million-fold amount of the final, effector hormone (e.g., hydrocortisone) which has global and drastic effects on the organism's total physiological responses.

The nervous system is organized into two major categories: the *central nervous system* or *CNS* and the *peripheral nervous system* (figure 13). The central nervous system consists of the brain and its lateral extensions, the optic nerves and retinae, and the spinal cord. The peripheral nervous system is made up of the nerve pathways running from the base of the brain and the spinal cord out to the peripheral regions of the body where they innervate and receive signals from a wide variety of sensory receptors, muscles and effector organs. Within the CNS, aggregates of cell bodies of neurons (gray matter) are termed *nuclei;* groups of such cell bodies within the peripheral nervous system are referred to as *ganglia.*

THE PERIPHERAL NERVOUS SYSTEM

The peripheral nervous system has two main divisions: the *somatic nervous system* and the *autonomic nervous system*. The somatic system consists of spinal pathways which receive sensory input from outlying receptor organs, as well as the outgoing motor pathways innervating the *skeletal* or *voluntary musculature*. These efferent (motor) fibers are under conscious control and the effector muscles they subtend can be activated quite at will by messages sent down from the brain. The somatic nervous system also includes many monosynaptic and polysynaptic *reflex arcs*, the basic functional units of the nervous system. In a reflex arc system, a stimulus from the peripheral receptors such as the pain from burning one's hand on a hot stove are sent immediately to the spinal cord, where it is simultaneously relayed up to the higher brain centers for registry and integrated action as well as to spinal *interneurons* which connect to somatic efferent fibers and which automatically cause a reflexive jerking back of the burned hand to avoid further damage. This reflex occurs long before the brain has even received the message, let alone decided what to do about it. By the time one is aware of having burned one's hand, the reflexive response has long since yanked it out of harm's way. The well known patellar or knee reflex is another such reflex arc. Reflex arcs are *not* themselves under conscious control, unlike the motor pathways to the skeletal muscles, but they do involve those same voluntary muscles which are normally moved voluntarily.

The autonomic nervous system innervates the viscera and the involuntary *smooth muscle* which causes the heart to pump blood and the *sinoatrial node* or pacemaker which times and coordinates its contractions, the respiratory tract, the salivary and lacrimal glands, the muscles which move the iris of the eye, the bladder, and even the genitalia, sexual arousal and detumescence. The autonomic system is itself subdivided into the *sympathetic* and *parasympathetic systems*.

The sympathetic system consists of nerve pathways emerging bilaterally from each vertebra in the thoracic and lumbar regions of the spine—that region below the neck but above the sacral or "tailbone" vertebrae. Sympathetic nerves primarily innervate the viscera: the heart, respiratory tract, stomach and both small and large intestines, the liver, spleen, kidneys and bladder, the medulla of the adrenal glands, and the genitalia (figure 13A). The primary purpose of the sympathetic system is to respond to severe stress and threat to life or limb. It immediately prepares the organism for fighting or fleeing and the massive activation of the sympathetic system, either in response to a real, physical danger or merely to extreme emotional agitation and anxiety in itself severely stresses the organism. Sympathetic arousal of the adrenal medulla initiates the release of norepinephrine and epinephrine. This precipitates a marked increase in heart rate, blood pressure and peripheral vasoconstriction. Epinephrine also inhibits glycogen synthetase and activates glycogen phosphorylase, thus depleting liver and muscular glycogen reserves (see Light 1985). There is a concomitant rise in blood glucose levels. At the same time, severe stress causes a pituitary mediated (via corticotropin) release of clucocorticoids (steroids) mostly in the form of *hydrocortisone* (cortisol) (figure 14). This tends to conserve glycogen stores and reconverts glucose back into glycogen. On the other hand hydrocortisone catabolizes proteins and mobilizes amino acids for gluconeogenesis which again elevates blood glucose levels. Both epinephrine and hydrocortisol mobilize free fatty acids from the adipose stores (see Light 1985) and enhance beta-oxidation of fatty acids for energy. All of these effects prepare the organism for extreme, emergency action.

However, once the crisis subsides or has otherwise been resolved, the organism must be transformed from this extreme and under normal circumstances pathological state of arousal, and restored to a normal state of reasonably tranquil physiological activity. This is accomplished by the parasympathetic system. The parasympathetic system consists of autonomic fibers emerging from the cranial portion of the CNS, that is the mid- and hind-brain, as well as from the sacral vertebrae of the spinal cord. Afferent fibers uninterrupted by synapses bring messages from pressure- and chemosensitive receptor organs in the carotid sinus and carotid bodies and in the arch of the dorsal aorta. Whereas the sympathetic system prepares for flight or fighting, the parasympathetic is largely restorative and calming. The parasympathetic system innervates most of the same visceral organs as does the sympathetic system, and the two are generally antagonistic to each other.

The three divisions of the peripheral nervous system are also somewhat structurally different from each other (figure 13). In the somatic nervous system both afferent and efferent fibers run in unbroken lines between the spinal cord and the receptor and effector organs, respectively. That is, no synapses occur between the periphery and the spinal portion of the CNS. In some cases, such as in the limbs, single nerve pathways are over a meter long before they synapse with spinal interneurons. The

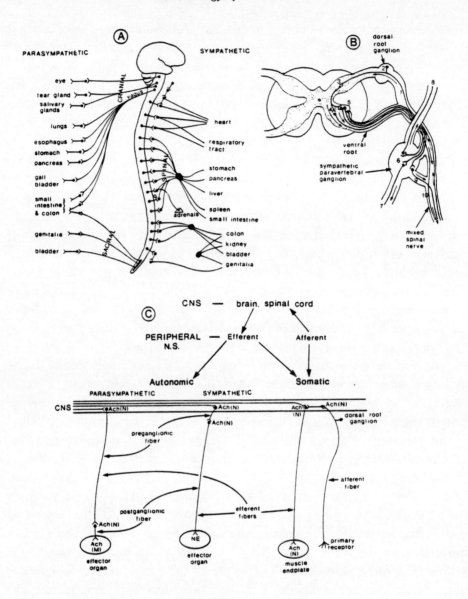

Figure 13
Somatic and Autonomic Nervous System

A. Relationship between the spinal sympathetic and the cranial and sacral para-sympathetic systems. The two systems act in opposition to each other; the sympathetic system generally readies the organism for combat or flight and the parasympathetic system typically acts in a restorative fashion. B. Cross-section of the spinal cord and associated nerve tracts, showing the relationship between the somatic and sympathetic systems. An afferent somatic signal (1) passes through the dorsal root ganglion [the cell body of this fiber lies within the ganglion] at (2) and enters the dorsal horn of the spinal gray matter where it is transmitted to one or more interneurons (3). A somatic efferent response is generated (4) which travels out to the skeletal muscles within the mixed spinal nerve (10). Interneurons also synapse with sympathetic fibers (5) and efferent signals enter the paravertebral ganglion (6) where they are relayed to the viscera (7), along the sympathetic chain to higher and lower paravertebral ganglia (8), or out to peripheral effector organs (9) such as the arrectori pilorum (the muscles which erect the body hairs and cause "goose bumps"). C. The relationship of all the components of the nervous system to one another. Afferent signals come in to the CNS from the peripheral somatic receptors. Efferent messages are sent out along both the somatic and autonomic systems. There are no synapses within the somatic system between the CNS and the peripheral receptors or effectors. Both branches of the autonomic system have a synaptic ganglion between the CNS and the distal effector organ. The preganglionic fibers of the sympathetic pathways are very short; those of the parasympathetic system are extremely long. The situation is reversed with respect to the postganglionic fibers. Acetylcholine is the neurotransmitter released at all synapses of the somatic and autonomic systems and their spinal interneuron connections, with the single exception that norepinephrine is released at the postganglionic terminals of the sympathetic pathways and their effector organs. All of these cholinergic receptors are nicotinic with the exception of the parasympathetic postganglionic synapse with the effector organs: here the receptors are muscarinic (see text). Ach = acetylcholine; NE = norepinephrine; N = nicotinic receptors; M = muscarinic receptors. Cholinergic receptors within the brain itself (not figured here) are mostly muscarinic, about which more later.

---

cell bodies of the afferent fibers lie outside the spinal cord itself in the *dorsal root ganglia* (figure 13); the dendrites of these nerves are located peripherally near the sensory receptor organs and the axonal tips synapse with interneurons within the spinal cord.

Most lower somatic motor neurons bear one or more *recurrent collaterals* which branch off from the axon and synapse with special interneurons known as *Renshaw cells* (figure 15). These Renshaw cells form multiple synapses with a number of somatic efferent (motor) fibers, including the one innervating them, via recurrent collaterals. When the motor fiber is fired the action potential sweeps down both the axon and the recurrent collateral side branch. The Renshaw cell is thus triggered into action along with the motor fiber. Where the Renshaw cell synapses with the motor neurons, however, the strongly inhibitory neurotransmitter glycine may be released into the synaptic cleft, causing the postsynaptic membrane to be hyperpolarized. This inhibition counteracts the original stimulus which generates it and the more a given motor pathway is stimulated into firing, the more it is automatically inhibited from firing at the same time. Renshaw cells also innervate the motor fibers subtending opposing muscle groups from the one being activated by a given pathway. In such cases, the Renshaw cells may release an excitatory neurotransmitter such as

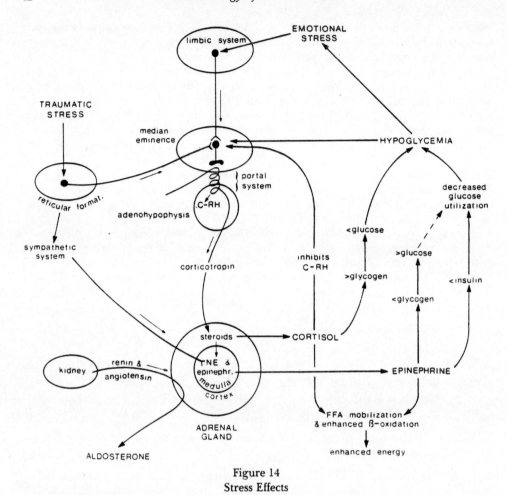

Figure 14
Stress Effects

NE = norepinephrine; FFA = free fatty acids; C—RH = corticotropin releasing hormone (factor); > = increase; < = decrease. Modified and expanded from a drawing by Bowman & Rand 1980.

acetylcholine,[20] and this causes a partial contraction of the opposing muscles. Thus, flexor muscles tend to partially contract in response to the strong contraction of the corresponding extensors. In this way a proper balance is maintained between opposing muscle groups during normal physical activity which prevents severe cramps and seizures that would otherwise occur.

---

[20]Although recent research suggests that there may be many exceptions to this rule (for example, Hökfelt et al., 1984), neurons release only one given transmitter at their axon terminals. The receptors of a given neuron can, however, be activated by a different transmitter from the one it releases at its own terminals. And different Renshaw cells can release different neurotransmitters.

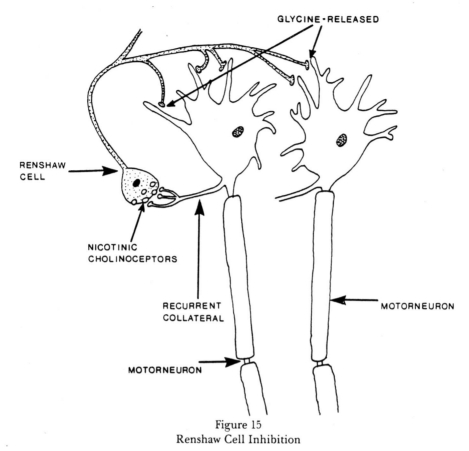

Figure 15
Renshaw Cell Inhibition

Lower motor neurons each give off a recurrent collateral within the spinal cord that synapses with an inhibitory interneuron called a Renshaw cell. The axon terminals of the Renshaw cell forms synapses with several lower motor neurons, thus creating a system of negative feedback loops. Activity from a lower motor neuron thus activates the Renshaw cell which in turn inhibits the motor neuron which excited it. The Renshaw cells not only inhibit the motor neurons which excite them; they also inhibit the inhibitory neurons (not shown) impinging on antagonistic motor neurons. This disinhibition of antagonistic motor neurons amounts to indirect stimulation. Antagonistic skeletal muscles are thus brought into play whenever agonistic muscles are activated. This exerts a modulating effect on the original action.

In both divisions of the autonomic system efferent pathways to the visceral or peripheral effector organs are interrupted by a single synapse located within extraspinal ganglia known as *prevertebral* and *paravertebral ganglia,* depending upon their position relative to the spinal cord. The fibers running from the spinal cord to the extraspinal ganglion in both the sympathetic and parasympathetic systems are called *preganglionic* fibers or pathways; those running from the ganglia to the effector organs are the *postganglionic* pathways. Like somatic motor neurons, autonomic preganlionic fibers give off axonal collaterals which synapse with Renshaw-like inhibitory interneurons which dampen the effects of preganglionic stimulation on the postganglionic fibers. Dopamine is the transmitter released by the interneurons. In the sympathetic system the pregangli-onic fibers are quite short relative to the much longer postganglionic fibers, and the ganglia between the two lie fairly close to the spinal cord. In the parasympathetic system the preganglionic fibers are extremely long and the postganglionic fibers very short; the ganglia lie far distally near the effector organ.

Acetylcholine is the neurotransmitter bridging the synapses between the afferent neurons of the somatic system and in many of the spinal interneurons (excepting certain Renshaw and substance P releasing pain cells), as well as between interneurons and the efferent fibers and between the efferent pathways and the *neuromuscular endplates* which innervate the skeletal muscles. Acetylcholine is also involved in neurotransmission between all of the synapses in both divisions of the autonomic system, except for the junction between the postganglionic fibers and the effector organs of the sympathetic system. In the last case, norepinephrine is released by the postganglionic neurons to activate the receptors of the various end organs.

Postsynaptic receptor sites which are activated by acetylcholine are referred to as *cholinoceptive* receptors. Neurons which release acetylcho-line from the axon terminals are *cholinergic neurons.*[21] *Nicotine and related cholinomimetic* alkaloids mimic the action of acetylcholine in many of these receptors, which are appropriately enough called *nicotinic receptors.* Low doses of nicotine mimic the action of acetylcholine on such recep-tors whereas larger doses block the response. Part of the reason for these apparently contradictory actions appears to result from the long-term postsynaptic depolarization generated by high concentrations of nicotine. This may cause a "current sink" into which local circuit charges bleed from peripheral membrane areas, further inhibiting membrane activation. The possible allosteric effects that partial agonists such as nicotine may exert upon these receptors may also be involved. This phenomenon is pursued in some detail in Volume 4, which deals with the combined interactions of nicotine and alcohol upon the body and psyche of humans

---

[21]Neurons which release acetylcholine from their axon terminals are *cholinergic;* those which release dopa-mine are dopaminergic, or norepinephrin are *adrenergic,* and those releasing serotonin are *serotoninergic.*

(Light, in press, Volume 4). Nicotinic receptors occur at all cholinergic synapses within the somatic nervous system, including those between the efferent fibers and the neuromuscular endplates (figure 13). They are also found in all autonomic ganglia. The cholinoceptive sites of all spinal interneurons are also nicotinic.

Some cholinergic neurons also respond to *muscarine*—a potent psychoactive alkaloid found in the poisonous fly agaric mushroom, *Amanita muscaria*—but not to nicotine; the receptors on such neurons are *muscarinic receptors* (see also Light, in press, Volume 4). In the peripheral nervous system they occur primarily in the postsynaptic membranes between the parasympathetic postganglionic fibers and their effector end-organs. The vast majority of cholinoceptive receptors within the brain itself are muscarinic, although nicotinic receptors also occur there. About 25% of all neurons in the cerebral cortex respond to acetylcholine with excitement; these are mostly muscarinic. Many of the acetylcholine-releasing axon terminals within the cortex originate in the reticular formation and are part of the reticular activating system (Bowman & Rand 1980) [see also below]. More than half of the spontaneously active hippocampal neurons are muscarinic and respond to acetylcholine with excitement. This is also true for more than 80% of the neurons of the caudate nucleus, although a few are inhibited by acetylcholine. Both muscarinic and nicotinic receptors occur in the thalamus, at least some of which probably originate in the reticular formation. Within the hypothalamus there are equal numbers of excitatory and inhibitory cholinoceptive neurons. And more than 50% of the neurons in the brainstem, especially in the pons and medulla oblongata are cholinergic; of these, about 57% are excited and the rest are inhibited by acetylcholine (all of these figures from Bowman & Rand 1980). Excitatory responses to acetylcholine are mediated by both nicotinic and muscarinic receptors, whereas inhibitory responses are mediated primarily by muscarinic receptors.

Norepinephrine, and not acetylcholine, is released by the sympathetic postganglionic fibers and the respective postsynaptic receptors are adrenergic; they do not respond to acetylcholine, nicotine or muscarine. There are two types of noradrenergic receptors:

(1) *alpha-adrenergic sites*—these sites are extremely responsive to norepinephrine; they cause contraction of most smooth muscle, except in intestinal smooth muscle where they cause relaxation.

(2) *beta-adrenergic sites*—these sites are less reactive to norepinephrine

than are the alpha-adrenergic sites, and adenylate cyclase and cAMP play a major role in mediating the actions of these receptor subtypes. Beta-adrenergic receptors are divided into two types based upon their actions upon specific muscle systems: (a) β_1-receptors cause contraction of intestinal smooth muscle and increase cardiac rate and output; (b) β_2-receptors cause relaxation in the smooth muscle of the bronchii, uterus and periphereal blood vessels. Specific β_1-receptor antagonists (the so-called "beta-blockers") are very effective in treating cardiac arrhythmias and angina.

Finally, dopaminergic (dopamine-activated) receptors are highly concentrated in the basal ganglia, hypothalamus, and in the ventral portion of the mesencephalon (see below), and they are also associated with certain inhibitory interneurons within the autonomic ganglia. Dopaminergic receptors are also divided into two subgroups: (a) D_1-receptors which are activated via a second-messenger system involving adenylate cyclase, and (b) D_2-receptors which directly open ionic gates. This brings us now to a consideration of the higher regions of the central nervous system, namely the brain and brainstem.

THE CENTRAL NERVOUS SYSTEM

The central nervous system in vertebrate animals begins as two parallel ridges of neural ectoderm which emerge from the uppermost or dorsal surface of the developing embryo (see Light, in press, Volume 4). These two ridges soon fuse along their lengths, forming an elongated, hollow *neural tube.* As development proceeds a series of swollen chambers connected by constrictions form along the neural tube (figure 16), dividing the presumptive CNS into three major sections. Early in the embryonic development and phylogenetic evolution[22] of this system the tube is divided into the *prosencephalon, mesencephalon* and *rhombencephalon,* corresponding to the *forebrain, midbrain* and *hindbrain,* respectively. The prosencephalon then subdivides into the *telencephalon* and the

---

[22]The nineteenth-century German naturalist-philosopher Ernst Haeckel proposed the famous axiom that "ontogeny [embryonic development] recapitulates phylogeny [the sequences of changes occurring in a related but diverse group of organisms during the evolutionary history of that group]." Although this phenomenon is by no means as all-pervasive as was once thought, it is true enough to remain well established as a fundamental principle in biology. It is evidenced in such things as the development of transient gills and tails in the growing embryos of mammals (including humans) reflecting the evolutionary changes which occured in the evolution of vertebrates from ancestral fishes through amphibians and reptiles to modern mammals.

diencephalon, and the rhombencephalon gives rise to the *metencephalon* and the *myelencephalon* (figure 16A).

The telencephalon develops into two large, side-by-side chambers termed the *first and second ventricles.* The enclosing walls of these chambers are destined to become the two cerebral hemispheres of the adult brain—the portion of the CNS associated with consciousness, learning and reasoning. The floor of the two ventricles of the telencephalon gives rise to the *basal ganglia* of the adult brain which comprise the *limbic system*, involved in the experience and regulation of affect or emotion. Projecting anteriorly (forward) from the cerebral hemispheres are two *olfactory bulbs* which retain a prominent sensory role in the lower vertebrates (including many mammals), but which in man have lost much of their former function. The olfactory bulbs and their attached *olfactory tubercles* (figures 16 and 17) remain an integral part of the limbic system in man, however, and are partly responsible for the powerful emotional senses of *déjà vu* which we all experience from time to time associated with odors which are either real or "hallucinatory" and which remind us very strongly of some early experience which we can never really quite "place."

The diencephalon encloses the *third ventricle* of the brain. The side walls of the diencephalon comprise the *thalamus*,[23] *the floor of that structure becomes the hypothalamus*, and the roof the *epithalamus* from which emerge three glandular bodies: the *paraphysis, epiphysis* or *pineal organ*, and the *parapineal* or *parietal organ*. A prominent ventral (downward) outpocket of the diencephalon is known as the *infundibulum* (see above page 34 and figure 16A); it will form the posterior lobe of the pituitary gland—the neurohypophysis. The anterior pituitary or adenohypophysis derives from Rathke's pouch which pinches off from the roof of the embryonic mouth and migrates to the infundibulum with which it fuses (figures 12 and 16). The *optic chiasma* also arises within the hypothalamus just anterior to the pituitary complex; this structure marks the point at which the optic fibers from the eyeballs enter the main part of the brain, half of the fibers from each tract crossing over into the opposite side of the brain. The optic nerves and retinae of the eyes are themselves formed from direct outpockets of the diencephalon (figure 16A–B) and

---

[23]This refers to both the two entire side walls of the diencephalon, which also is incorporated as part of the limbic system (figures 18 and 19). The thalami are derived from the diencephalon, whereas the other basal ganglia develop from the floor of the telencephalon. See also footnote 27.

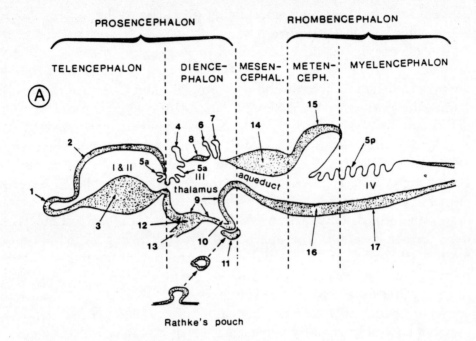

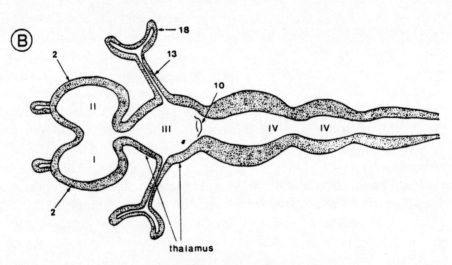

Figure 16
Primitive/Embryonic Divisions of the Brain

A. Median longitudinal section through embryonic brain. The three major divisions of the brain, the prosencephalon, mesencephalon and rhombencephalon, correspond to the forebrain, midbrain and hindbrain, respectively. 1 = olfactory tubercle; 2 = cerebral hemispheres; 3 = floor of telencephalon which gives rise to the paired basal ganglia of the adult brain; 4 = paraphysis, a structure of obscure function; 5a = anterior choroid plexus; 5p = posterior choroid plexus; 6 = parapineal (parietal organ); 7 = epiphysis (pineal body); 8 = epithalamus; 9 = hypothalamus; 10 = infundibulum; 11 = adenohypophysis and pars intermedia, derived from Rathke's pouch; 12 = optic chiasma; 13 = optic tract; 14 = tectum; 15 = cerebellum; 16 = pons; 17 = medulla oblongata.

B. Overhead or dorsal view of plane section through the embryonic brain. The numbers are the same as in figure 16A, above; 18 = developing retinal cup of the eye, a structure deriving directly as a lateral outgrowth of the diencephalon. Roman numerals indicate the various ventricles of the brain in both figures. The prosencephalon = the forebrain; mesencephalon = midbrain; rhombencephalon = hindbrain.

---

are thus true extensions of the brain. Posterior to the infundibulum, the hypothalamus gives rise to two side-by-side ventral protuberances known as the *mammillary bodies.* These nuclei are prominently involved in memory functions and in the expression of rage.

The previously mentioned pineal and parietal organs derived from the epithalamus appear to have served in ancient vertebrates[24] as a functional pair of median eyes; this median pair was in addition to the pair of lateral eyes derived from the left and right thalami exhibited by all vertebrates who have not secondarily lost them (as in some cave-dwelling fishes). The pineal organ persists in higher vertebrates (including the mammals) as a glandular structure with light-receptive endocrine functions. Fibers from the optic tracts go directly to the pineal body in modern vertebrates. This organ is directly influenced by the seasonal variations in daylight to darkness ratios and it regulates the release of hypophyiotropic hormones from the hypothalamus. The pineal body thus plays a paramount role in determining the onset and duration of the reproductive or estrous cycle in modern vertebrates, including mammals.

The brain is mostly surrounded by thick walls of neural tissue except for two regions: the junction between the roof of the telencephalon and that of the anterior part of the diencephalon (the epithalamus) and the roof of much of the *fourth ventricle*—the expanded part of the neural cavity lying behind the third ventricle. In these two regions is found a

---

[24]Modern lampreys possess a pair of median eyelike structures of which the one derived from the pineal organ is the dominent element. These jawless fishlike animals are the living remnants of the earliest class of vertebrates, the Agnatha. The earliest agnathans were the *ostracoderms* which flourished in Cambrian and Ordovician freshwater habitats in Colorado and Greenland nearly 500 million years ago. These creatures possessed two well-developed median eyes, as did certain later *placoderms,* an extinct class of fishlike vertebrates. The living rhynchocephalian, *Sphenodon* or the tuatara of New Zealand, represents an ancient reptilian lineage which long predates even the earliest of dinosaurs. The tuatara bears a median functional eye derived from the parapineal body.

thin, highly complex and folded tissue rich in blood vessels—the *anterior* and *posterior choroid plexi* (singular, *plexus*), respectively. The choroid plexi are regions in which the exchange of materials occurs between the blood and the fluid of the CNS ventricles or the *cerebrospinal fluid.* These two systems become extremely important later on in our discussion of the blood-brain barrier and the access of xenobiotics or foreign substances such as drugs and alcohol to the brain itself.

Within the mesencephalon or midbrain region, the central cavity, which is well developed and expansive in lower vertebrates (the several fish classes and the amphibians), but which is very narrow and restricted in the reptiles, birds and mammals, is termed the *aqueduct of Sylvius.* This aqueduct connects the third and fourth ventricles. The thickened roof of neural tissue overlying the aqueduct of Sylvius is called the *tectum.* It gives rise to four small, rounded mounds known as the *corpora quadrigemina.* The anterior two side-by-side mounds are the *superior colliculi;* the posterior pair comprises the *inferior colliculi.* The superior and inferior colliculi help to integrate visual and auditory signals, respectively, and they function in pupillary and auditory reflexes.

The roof of the metencephalon gives rise to the *cerebellum,* a complex brain center involved in the coordination and regulation of motor activity and in the maintainance of balance and posture. It is affected by many psychotropic drugs, including alcohol, and this response is responsible for the *ataxia* or loss of motor coordination seen in intoxication. The floor of the metencephalon gives rise to the *pons,* which is a pathway for ascending and descending nerve tracts between the brain and spinal cord. Synapses between fibers descending from the cerebral cortex and tracts from the cerebellum also occur in the pons. The *reticular formation* (figure 21) of the mid- and hindbrain also passes through the pons, as well as through the lower lying *medulla oblongata* which occupies the myelencephalon. The myelencephalon is essentially an expanded version of the spinal cord, but it contains in addition to the reticular formation pathways, important nerve centers involved in the control of blood pressure, heart rate, respiration, temperature, and vomiting.

The description of the brain thus far pertains to the primitive brain structure exhibited by lower vertebrates and the early embryonic stages of higher vertebrates. In man, the primitive structures just described undergo drastic changes in the configuration of these elements (figure 17). Because humans walk upright, the orientation of the brain structures is from top to bottom, rather than fore to aft as in quadrupedal animals.

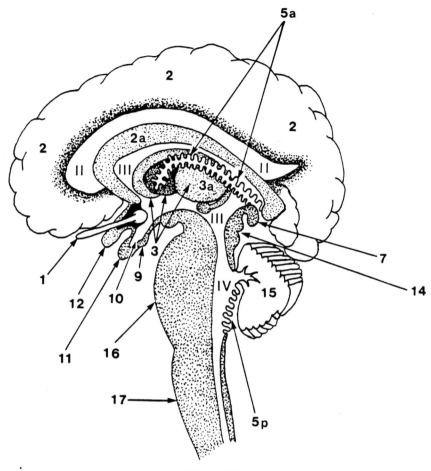

Figure 17
Median Longitudinal Section of Human Brain I

In this figure of the adult human brain, the basic structures depicted in figure 16 are shown here as collapsed back upon the brainstem with the cerebral hemispheres flanking the diencephalon on each side. The thalamus is now restricted to two reduced ganglia flanking the now considerably compressed third ventricle. The other basal ganglia are derived from the floor of the telencephalon. The olfactory bulbs and tubercles are considerably reduced from the embryonic condition and they are allied and interconnected with the amygdala of the limbic system. The numbers are the same as in figure 16, except that 3 = the basal ganglia including the thalamus, and 3a = the thalamus itself. The tectum (14) is shown here as the four mounded nuclei of the corpora quadrigemina.

The brainstem has become a vertical mushroom-like structure crowned by the hypothalamus and paired thalami of the diencephalon. The cortically derived (from the floor of the telencephalon) basal ganglia of the limbic system surround the diencephalon. The paired lateral cerebral ventricles (I & II) project laterally from the level of the diencephalon, and are themselves enclosed by the massive, convoluted tissue masses of the two cerebral hemispheres.

In very early and primitive vertebrates the telencephalon is closely associated with the development of olfactory lobes, and the cerebral hemispheres in such animals are primarily concerned with integrating and processing olfactory sensations. This is the case with modern lampreys. The cerebral cortex at this stage of evolutionary development is known as the *paleocortex* or *paleopallium* ("ancient" cortex). In higher vertebrates such as amphibians and reptiles the paleocortex is restricted to the lower sidewalls and floor of the telencephalon and the attached olfactory bulbs. This paleocortical region is the one which gives rise to the basal ganglia of the limbic system in reptiles and the more advanced mammals. Above the paleocortex and towards the center of the cerebral hemispheres lies the *archicortex* or *archipallium* ("old" cortex). This region gives rise to the *hippocampus* in mammals by a recurved folding of the inner medial part of the temporal lobes (figures 18 and 19). The paleocortex and archicortex and their derived structures are commonly referred to as the "reptilian brain." They are closely associated with emotional behavior in the higher mammals.

The advanced brains of mammals and particularly of humans are thus arranged in a series of concentric shells, with the evolutionarily and embryologically most advanced and recently differentiated shells encapsulating the earlier and more primitive portions. The limbic system from the reptilian brain together with the hypothalamus from the floor of the diencephalon are involved in the experience and expression of emotional states, particularly of rage and aggression. These primitive functions are modified, channeled and inhibited by the surrounding, outer shell of the neocortex. This point will become very important later in this section in our discussion of the effects of alcohol and other psychotropic drugs upon the CNS.

The cerebral hemispheres in humans cover the entire brain as paired, massive, and highly convoluted globes which have grown forward, laterally and rearward to cap the diencephalon and midbrain region like a huge mushroom (figures 18 and 19). The outermost few centimeters of the cerebral cortex is gray matter consisting of densely intertwined cell bodies of more than 12 billion or so neurons. Beneath the outermost portion lie the massive myleinated fibers and pathways of the white matter of the brain. The surface convolutions—the *gyri* or ridges and *sulci* or the valleys between the gyri—occur only in advanced mammals.

Such surface contortions allow for a very greatly expanded surface area and can thus accommodate the exponentially increased numbers of cortical neurons necessary to such animals as the higher mammals, and especially of man. Despite the fascinating and detailed story presented by the neocortex with respect to learning, memory and data retrieval and the phenomenon of lateralization (right- and left-handedness) of such functions as logic and reason, intuition and spatial perception, language, and the like, space does not permit further discussion of that most intricate and awe-inspiring of organic systems. Those details are neither relevant nor immediately necessary to understanding how ethanol and other drugs affect human cognition, perception, and affective (emotional) behavior.

A rather detailed discussion of the lower regions of the CNS from the limbic system on down is required, however, since it is here that most of the effects of drugs are manifested upon the CNS. Figure 19 shows the arrangement of these structures within the human brain and brainstem. Beneath the neocortex lies a massive tract of myelinated fibers running sideways from one cerebral hemisphere to the other. This tract, known as the *corpus callosum* connects the two hemispheres and allows for the integrated functioning of the right and left halves of the brain. Without the corpus callosum, for example, we would not be able to think or talk about a painting or musical work. Nor could we describe a sensation occurring on the left side of the body to another person.[25] In fact, we would have two very separate and individual consciousnesses, with neither being even aware of the other's existence![26]

Beneath the corpus callosum the paired basal ganglia derived from the paleocortex form a complex dome which surrounds the third ventricle and the underlying hypothalamus (figures 18D and 19). The adjective *limbic* refers to the ringlike structure or limbus formed by the basal ganglia around the top of the brainstem. The limbic system contains

---

[25]Events on the left side of the body are primarily communicated to the right half of the brain. Since language is mainly associated with the left cerebral hemisphere, it would not be possible to integrate the experience with language.

[26]Actually, *all* of the connections between the right and left halves of the brain would have to be severed to cause the complete splitting of consciousnesses I have described. This includes not only the corpus callosum, but also the anterior commissure, optic chiasma, the *massa intermedia* which connects the right and left thalami, the habenular commissure, and the corpora quadrigemina. Such *split-brain preparations* have been well studied in laboratory animals and are also known clinically in humans because of the radical surgery required to control certain severe cases of otherwise intractable epilepsy or other organic brain disorder. Split-brain patients behave quite normally, except that they have two quite independent awarenesses and they often learn a task or function with one side of the body that they cannot communicate to the other.

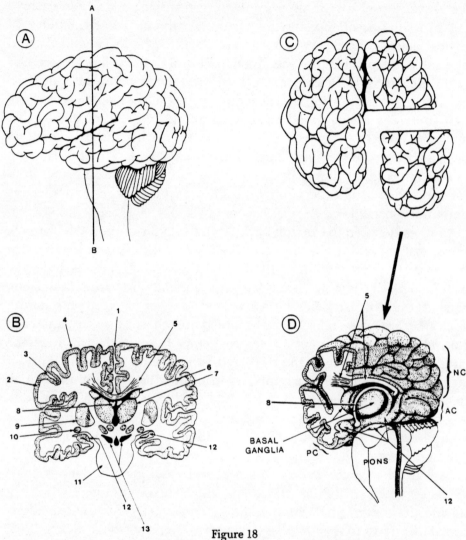

Figure 18
Human Brain: Cross and Mediotransverse Sections

A. Left side view of human brain. Line A–B indicates the plane of the section shown in B. B. Cross section through human brain along line A–B in figure 18A. The corpus callosum connects the two cerebral hemispheres and forms a roof over the third ventricle. The two thalami form the side walls of the third ventricle; they and the fornix, which connects the mammillary bodies of the hypothalamus to the hippocampus, are shown in cross-section. The relationships between the third ventricle, thalamus, and the basal ganglia (caudate nucleus, corpus striatum shown here) and the hippocampus are figured. The substantia nigra sends dopamine releasing fibers to the thalamus and corpus striatum. Excessive loss of neurons in the substantia nigra gives rise to Parkinson's syndrome. C. Dorsal view of brain showing the planes of section for the right posterior quarter figured in 18D. D. The posterior right quarter of the brain showing both a cross-sectional plane and the surface which forms the wall of the longitudinal fissure. The hippocampus is formed by a reflexive folding of the lower lateral and lower posterior edge of the cortex (compare figures D and B). This fold runs antero-posteriorly and flexes to the midline of the brain as it moves rearward. The corpus callosum is shown in both a cross-sectional and longitudinal planes. 1 = longitudinal fissure; 2 = complexly folded gray matter of the cerebral cortex; 3 = sulcus; 4 = gyrus; 5 = corpus callosum; 6 = caudate nucleus; 7 = thalamus; 8 = fornix; 9 = corpus striatum [= globus pallidus and putamen] or lentiform nucleus; 10 = tail of caudate nucleus; 11 = pons; 12 = hippocampus; 13 = substantia nigra. AC = archicortex; NC = neocortex; PC = paleocortex.

---

three large, paired nuclei: the *caudate nucleus, putamen* and *globus pallidus;* the putamen and globus pallidus collectively form the *corpus striatum* or *lentiform nucleus.*[27] These nuclei receive fibers from both the higher and lower brain centers, and together with the thalamus and cerebellum are important centers for motor coordination and activity. For example, dopaminergic (dopamine-releasing) neurons from the *substantia nigra* — a center in the anterior midbrain located just below the mammillary bodies (figure 19) — connect with the corpus striatum and thalamus where they exert an inhibitory effect. These neurons are continually dying throughout the adult life of the individual and a person of seventy or so years will have lost nearly half of the original neurons contained in the substantia nigra. As these neurons die a proportional amount of the inhibition upon the striatum and thalamus is lost. In most cases this cell loss is insufficient to cause any noticeable difficulties. However, some persons who have suffered an additional heavy loss of these neurons from such causes as influenza or other viral infections involving neuron death may lose a critical, threshold number of these neurons at some point in middle or late life. When this occurs the inhibitory release upon the thalamus and corpus striatum is enough to produce the progressively worse gross tremors and loss of motor control characteristic of Parkinson's syndrome. This follows because the striatum and thalamus are normally in a constant state of spontaneous activity which is normally under the control of the basal ganglia and thalamus. The net effect of massive neuronal death within the substantia nigra is that the corpus striatum and thalamus experience the effect of diminished levels of dopamine at the synaptic junctions (see also discussion below on schizophrenia and

---

[27]The term *basal ganglia* is restricted by some authors to just the caudate nucleus and corpus striatum; other writers also include the thalamus and amygdala under this term.

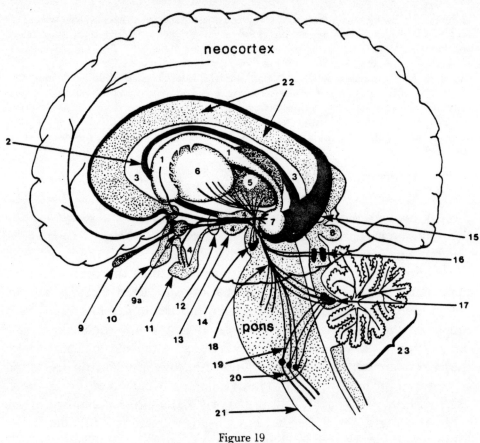

Figure 19
Human Brain: Median Longitudinal Section II

1 = caudate nucleus; 2 = fornix; 3 = third ventricle; 4 = hypothalamus; 5 = thalamus; 6 = corpus striatum (= putamen and globus pallidus); 7 = amygdala; 8 = pineal gland; 9 = olfactory bulb; 9a = olfactory tubercle; 10 = optic chiasma; 11 = pituitary (adenohypophysis); 12 = medial forebrain bundle; 13 = mammillary body; 14 = substantia nigra; 15 = hippocampus; 16 = raphe nuclei; 17 = locus coeruleus; 18 = ascending tracts from locus coeruleus; 19 = inter-connecting nerves between locus coeruleus and ascending and descending tracts; 20 = descending tracts from locus coeruleus; 21 = medulla oblongata; 22 = corpus callosum; 23 = cerebellum.

phenothiazine therapy). Parkinson's disease is often treated by adminis-tration of *levodopa* or *L-dopa*, a precursor of dopamine (see above, figure 9B), which to some extent compensates for the effective lack of dopamine.

    The caudate nucleus also connects the anterior hypothalamus and olfactory septal region to the paired *amygdala* located next to the hippo-campus on either side of the brain. The amygdala are involved in the maintainence of emotional control—particularly with the expression of hypothalamically-induced rage. The medial portion of the amygdala

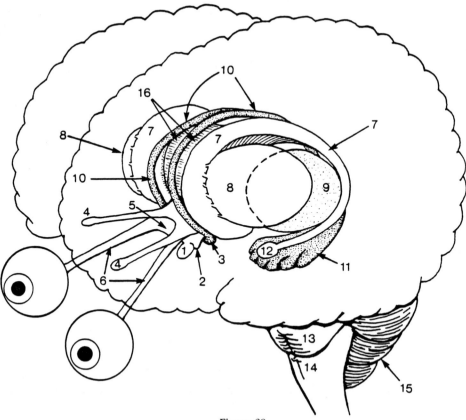

Figure 20
Basal Ganglia (Limbic System)

1 = adenohypophysis; 2 = neurohypophysis; 3 = left mammillary body; 4 = olfactory bulbs; 5 = optic chiasma; 6 = optic tracts; 7 = caudate nuclei (left and right); 8 = corpus striatum (= putamen and globus pallidus); 9 = left thalamus; 10 = fornix; 11 = hippocampus; 12 = amygdala; 13 = pons; 14 = medulla oblongata; 15 = cerebellum; 16 = interthalamic commissure (massa intermedia). Modified from The Brain: A User's Manual, 1982.

appears to inhibit hypothalamic aggression, whereas the basolateral portion excites hypothalamic aggression. In general, the hypothalamus appears to be involved in the *expression* of emotion, whereas the limbic system is concerned with the *experience* of emotion. Animals which have had their cortical and amygdaloid control over the hypothalamus surgically removed will exhibit violent rage to very slight tactile stimulation. In such cases, the animal responds to almost any minor sensation with an uncontrolled rage reaction. Because the rages are not directed at any particular target, but are rather random attacks at almost any object, this type of aggression is termed *sham rage*. There appears to be little or no emotional *experience* of rage during such an episode, but merely the overt and violent expression of rage.

The hippocampus is also involved in emotional control, as well as in learning and memory. It is especially concerned with learning situations based upon fear. It is connected to the mammillary bodies and other hypothalamic nuclei by the paired *fornix* (figures 19 and 20). Damage to the mammillary bodies tends to render otherwise ferocious animals quite docile and emotionally placid. The rage produced by specific lesions in the amygdala appears to result from the resulting release of inhibition upon the mammillary bodies. Wernicke-Korsakoff syndrome (see Volume 1 of this series; Light 1985) involves lesions in the mammillary bodies, thalamus and also the hippocampus which result from the combined effects of thiamine deficiency and the cytotoxic actions of alcohol. The lesions in the mammillary bodies may be associated with the passivity and indifference seen in such patients (who typically have a long, premorbid history of fighting and assault). The damage to the thalamus and hippocampus results in the severe loss of memory involving both retrograde and anterograde amnesia exhibited by such persons.

Emotional experience and expression thus involves a complex interaction between the hippocampus and associated areas of the cortex (the *cingulate gyrus* and the *hippocampal (dentate) gyrus* and *uncus*),[28] the thalamus and associated basal ganglia, the hypothalamic centers and the mammillary bodies, and the cerebral neocortex. This is known as the Papez circuit. Signals from the hypothalamus regarding pain, pleasure, thirst, hunger, sexual desire and satiety are routed via the thalamus to the higher cortex and the hippocampus and amygdala. These nuclei regulate the expression of these needs and emotional states and are themselves regulated by the higher cortex. The cortex, in turn, is affected by and modifies the signals coming from the hypothalamic centers and the encapsulating limbic system.

A complex set of diffusely interconnected neurons lies within the medulla oblongata and runs upward through the pons to end in the lower third of the thalamus on each side. This nerve network is called

---

[28]These portions of the neocortex are not figured. The dentate gyrus is that portion of the neocortical frontal lobe which directly overlies the contours of the coprus callosum. The dentate gyrus-uncus complex is that part of the temporal lobe lying adjacent to the hippocampus in each hemisphere.

the *reticular formation* (figure 21A). Major nerve tracts radiate from the top of the reticular formation and innervate all parts of the cerebral cortex. The reticular formation and associated pathways leading to the cerebral cortex are called the *reticular activating system* or *R.A.S.* This system is in a constant state of spontaneous activity and it sends impulses to the cortex which initiate and maintain a state of consciousness and alertness in the organism. The thalamus also mediates selective attention so that one can focus his attention upon a single situation. The thalamic-medullary reticular complex thus is the very seat of consciousness and of selective attention. In a related function, it is also the site where extraeneous information and nonsignificant stimuli are screened out. This system allows us to ignore a continually barking dog or the noise of highway traffic in our environment so that we can devote our attention to really important and novel signals, such as the sound of glass breaking or the alarm from a smoke detector. The phenomenon of screening background noise and other stimuli from consciousness is known as *accommodation*. Without this ability we would soon go quite mad under the continual bombardment of stimuli from all sources.

At periodic intervals serotoninergic neurons from two centers near the cerebellum known as the *raphe nuclei* (figure 21B) become active and release serotonin at their synapses with the R.A.S. This generates inhibitory postsynaptic potentials (see above, figure 10B) within the R.A.S., causing it to shut down much of its activity. This, in turn, allows the cerebral cortex to disengage, and as consciousness begins to recede, the organism lapses into the unconscious state we call sleep. Sleep consists of several, well-defined and alternating substates which will be simply summarized here as *deep sleep* and *rapid-eye-movement (REM) sleep*. Deep sleep is just that: a prolonged state of deep, coma-like unconsciousness during which the organism is unaware of anything at all. There are minor movements of the body from time to time during this stage of sleep as the position of the body is adjusted. These movements are due in part to the selective activity of descending fibers from the *locus coeruleus*, a nucleus of norepinephrine-releasing neurons located at the base of the cerebellum (figure 19). These descending fibers cause the minor activity of the lower body by their low-level activity during deep sleep.

At periodic intervals during the sleep cycle, the raphe nuclei back off and release part of their inhibition upon the R.A.S. At the same time, the signals from the locus coeruleus to the descending pathways are shut

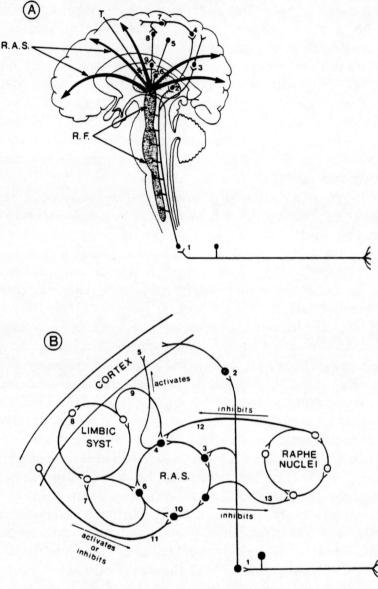

Figure 21
Reticular Activating System

A. Schematic figure showing relationships between the reticular formation, the limbic system, the cerebral cortex, and the reticular activating system which regulates consciousness and selective attention. The reticular activating system (R.A.S.) is always in a spontaneous state of excitement and activity. It therefore tends to maintain the cerebral cortex in a constant state of awareness. Stimuli coming into the CNS from peripheral sensory organs (1) act to further excite the R.A.S. by means of collateral fibers entering the reticular formation (R.F.) in the medulla oblongata and the pons. These same impulses go to the cerebral cortex via two routes: (a) information coming to the thalamus (2) is sorted out and relayed to the appropriate cortical areas (4) for further integration and processing (7,8, et cetera); (b) direct sensory pathways (3) convey the stimuli directly to the higher brain centers. The R.A.S. stimulates all areas of the cerebral cortex (bold radiating arrows) and is in turn both excited and inhibited by impulses from the higher cortex (7,8, et cetera). The higher cortex also mediates the activity of the limbic system (5 and 6) which also modulates the activity of the R.A.S. That portion of the R.A.S. formed by the lower portions of the thalamus (T) not only act to initiate or maintain consciousness, but also is responsible for the selective attention of the organism to specific stimuli or undertakings. Modified from Bowmand & Rand 1980.

B. Details of the interaction between the R.A.S., the cerebral cortex, the limbic system and the raphe nuclei in initiating and/or maintaining consciousness. Incoming messages (1) stimulate both the cerebral cortex (2) and the R.A.S. (3). The R.A.S. in turn activates the higher cortex (5) and the limbic system (7). The limbic system in turn acts upon the R.A.S. (6 and 9) in either an excitatory or inhibitory fashion, and is itself regulated by the higher cortex (8). The higher cortex also directly acts to excite or inhibit the limbic system (11). Consciousness is normally periodically terminated (as in sleep-wake cycles) by serotonin-releasing neurons in the raphe nuclei which inhibit the normally active state of the R.A.S. Neurons from the raphe nuclei inhibit the R.A.S. (12) and the raphe nuclei are themselves inhibited by the R.A.S. (13). Modified from Bowman & Rand 1980.

---

down, causing all bodily movements to cease. Additionally, however, fibers from the locus coeruleus to the R.A.S. become mildly active, and this together with the inhibitory release of the R.A.S. by the raphe nuclei results in mild to moderate arousal of the R.A.S. The consequent partial arousal of the consciousness activating system results in the semi-conscious state known as dreaming. Dreaming is associated with REM sleep. Although the consciousness is partially aroused and certain muscular movements of the face and eyes are prominent features of REM sleep (due to the partial activity of the ascending tracts of the locus coeruleus), the shut down of the descending tracts of the locus coeruleus inhibits all movements of the lower body during this stage.

Deep or *NREM* (*non-REM*) sleep thus depends upon a delicate balance between the amount of serotonin released by the raphe nuclei and the levels of norepinephrine from the locus coeruleus. Both neurotransmitters accumulate in the forebrain as they are released and forebrain levels of these agents correlate with the various rates of release and consequent stages of sleep and activity. If the locus coeruleus is destroyed, animals exhibit normal amounts of sleep, but REM sleep is not present. If an animal is deprived of sleep, an excessive amount of *rebound* REM sleep will ensue when sleep finally does occur. This rebound effect is seen in nearly all neurological functions involving neurotransmitters and their receptor sites in which the activity is artificially enhanced or repressed. The body attempts to maintain *homeostasis* or normal rates and levels of functioning, and when a neurotransmitter level is depressed, the organism will tend to increase its level of response to whatever amount is present. When normal concentrations are reestablished, then, an overshoot response is typically exhibited until the former, "normal" balance can be regained. The rebound REM sleep which occurs after sleep deprivation is associated with greatly increased levels of norepinephrine in the brain.

Many individuals with either situational or chronic neurotic conflict or tension experience mild to severe insomnia. This is due partly to the fact that cortical arousal tends to activate the R.A.S. and counter the effects of serotonin from the raphe nuclei (see the interactions shown in figure 21B). Either emotional tension generated within the limbic-hypothalamic axis or cortical activity generated by conscious focus upon a problem or situation can excite the R.A.S., which in turn can stimulate both the cortex and the limbic pathways. Psychological depression is the most common emotional problem in our society. It is very closely associated with insomnia and it results in the use of millions of dollars worth of prescription and over-the-counter sedative-hypnotics and soporific drugs annually. Much of the insomnia associated with depression is generated by simple psychic and cortical tension over one's job, life, or emotional state. However, a significant portion of such depression-mediated insomnia results from the inhibition of serotonin and norepinephrine associated with depressive disorders (about which, more below). Blood levels of serotonin do not correlate well with the effective brain levels of this neurotransmitter since neither serotonin, the catecholamines, nor acetylcholine can cross the blood-brain barrier. Instead, the amino acid precursors of these substances must be actively transported into the axonal endings, and the neurotransmitter subsequently synthesized within the terminal button by enzymes manufactured in the cell body of the neuron and later transported by axoplasmic flow into the terminal. Therefore the direct administration of intravenous serotonin cannot adequately compensate for any deficit of that substance in the R.A.S.

Tryptophan, the precursor amino acid for synthesizing serotonin, is a poor competitor relative to the other amino acids for the carrier proteins that carry these substances across neural membranes into axon terminals. However, insulin, in addition to packing sugar away as glycogen in the liver, also clears all amino acids except tryptophan from the blood by packing them away inside the cells of the body. A high carbohydrate meal before bedtime causes insulin to be released into the blood. Its competitors now absent, tryptophan is readily transported inside the appropriate axonal endings where it can be synthesized into serotonin. Because amino acids are the building blocks of proteins, avoidance of high protein meals in the evening will also result in lower levels of all amino acids. Milk also contains high concentrations of tryptophan, and enhancing tryptophan levels in the blood allows it to compete favorably with the other amino acids simply by its mass effect for the carrier proteins. A glass of milk at bedtime can often help to induce sleep.

Rage and aggression also involve the interplay between serotonin and norepinephrine. Eliciting sham rage by stimulation of the appropriate amygdaloid centers involves the release of norepinephrine. When the synthesis of this substance is blocked in experimental animals, the rage state induced will soon deplete the amount of norepinephrine released by the amygdala. Subsequent stimulation of the amygdala will fail to produce the rage response. The rage reaction is also enhanced or inhibited by drugs that elevate or decrease, respectively, the levels of catecholamines in general. Both serotonin and its precursor, 5-hydroxytryptophan (figure 9C) inhibit such rage responses. Furthermore, cholinergic systems also appear to be involved in rage reactions and aggression, particularly those muscarinic cholergic systems in the lateral hypothalamus.[29] In summary, rage and aggression appear to involve hyperactivity of certain amygdaloid neuronal groups, perhaps in part due to inadequate inhibition of the amygdala by serotonin. These responses are also associated with elevated norepinephrine levels in the forebrain and R.A.S., coupled with excessive acetylcholine activity at the level of the hypothalamus.

SUMMARY

The structural unit of the nervous system is the individual nerve cell or neuron, consisting of the cell body or soma typically bearing numerous dendrites which carry nervous signals from other neurons, and a long branched or unbranched axon, which transmits signals from the soma to other neurons down the line of transmission. Myelinated axons are wrapped in a concentric series of double membranes formed by

---

[29]It has been suggested (Bowman & Rand 1980) that the muscarine-bearing toadstools of the genus *Amanita* were used by Norse Viking warriors to induce a maniacal fury known as *berserk-rage* prior to their raiding sorties. Recall that the cholinoceptive receptors in the thalamus and limbic system are primarily muscarinic (see above, page 45).

specialized Schwann cells or oligodendrocytes. The white matter of the brain and spinal cord are densely packed with myelinated fibers; the gray matter refers to regions consisting primarily of nonmyelinated nerve cell bodies and their dendrites. In the peripheral nervous system, the myelin sheaths are interrupted at regular intervals, forming short gaps called nodes of Ranvier where the naked axons are in direct contact with the extracellular medium.

As is true for all animal cells, each neuron is surrounded by a plasma membrane composed of a phospholipid bilayer whose hydrophobic fatty acid tails point away from the intra- and extracellular water, and whose polar phosphate heads are attracted toward the watery environment inside and outside of the cell. Within this lipid bilayer are embedded a variety of proteins which serve as enzymes, structural units, ionic gates and their receptor sites, or as carrier molecules in the active or facilitated transport of other molecules across the membrane.

A constant resting potential, or difference in electrical charge between the inner and outer surfaces of the neural membrane, is characteristic of excitable membranes. Sodium ions (Na^+) are concentrated outside the neural membrane in the extracellular membrane, which is relatively impermeable to those ions. Potassiom ions (K^+) are concentrated on the inner side of the neural membrane. In this case, however, the membrane is readily permeable to K^+, which tend to leak to the outside down a concentration gradient. An active transport mechanism known as the sodium-potassium pump continuously forces K^+ back inside the nerve cell, however, in an energy-requiring process involving the conversion of ATP into ADP. As fast as the sodium-potassium pump transports the leaking K^+ back inside the cell, however, K^+ continues to leak to the exterior like water running through a sieve. Because K^+ leak to the exterior just slightly faster than they can be pumped back inside, a slight but constant negative charge is established relative to the exterior. This slight differential is the resting potential. ATP is generated by oxidative phosphorylation within the mitochondria of cells. Because of the enormous energy requirements of the sodium-potassium pump in maintaining the resting potential, a continuous supply of glucose and oxygen is critical to brain cells.

A typical nervous impulse is generated when an incoming stimulus causes the neural membrane to become suddenly permeable to Na^+. Specialized gates open up and Na^+ rush in through the now permeable membrane from the outside. This causes a change in membrane polarity and constitutes a nervous impulse signal. Graded impulses are created when incoming stimuli from other neurons cause polarity changes along the dendrites or cell body. The impulses vary with the strength of the incoming stimuli and they are algebraically summed over both distance and time. Excitatory graded potentials are created when generalized ionic gates open up in the postsynaptic membrane, causing Na^+ to rush inward and K^+ to exit—each ionic species travelling down its own concentration gradient. This results in a membrane depolarization. Inhibitory graded potentials are set up when the incoming stimuli cause specialized ionic gates only to open up; K^+ exits as before, but now negatively charged chloride ions (Cl^-) enter the cell in a rush. This results in an even greater negative charge inside the membrane relative to the outside: the membrane becomes hyperpolarized. This subtracts from the excitatory potentials (depolarizations) created in the same membrane system. It thus requires an increase in excitatory potentials to regain the lost excitatory state. If the sum total of all excitatory and inhibitory postsynaptic potentials reach the junction between the cell body and the axon—the so-called axon hillock—at a critical level of depolarization from the resting potential, an all-or-nothing action potential is generated.

Unlike the graded potentials, this is an invariant polarity reversal which propagates itself down the entire length of the axon. As Na^+ rush in through suddenly opened sodium channels, the reversal of electrical charge inside and outside the membrane causes adjacent portions of the membrane to lose electrons. This in turn causes a charge perturbation in those adjacent regions, resulting in the opening of still more sodium gates and causing a major polarity change in that region. The action potential is propagated more or less continuously along the lengths of nonmyelinated axons. However, myelinated axons exhibit an extremely rapid form of nervous transmission known as saltational conduction. Polarity reversals can only occur at the nodes of Ranvier where the naked axonal surfaces are in contact with the extracellular environment (the myelin sheaths are very efficient electrical insulators). As polarity destabilization occurs at a given node of Ranvier, electrical perturbations are created in the next node down the line, resulting in an influx of Na^+ at that point, which creates perturbations still further down the line, and so forth. Because of the phenomenon known as the absolute refractory period which follows each action potential spike, the action potential can only travel forward in a single direction. The action potential in

myelinated fibers thus travels not in a continuous series of closely adjacent spikes, but in a series of widely separated spikes occurring only at
the nodes of Ranvier. The potential thus bypasses the greatest part of the
axon's length, jumping instead from node to node. Because the distance
travelled is so much less than the actual length of the axon (which may be
a meter or more in some cases), the nervous impulse can propagate itself
extremely rapidly.

As the action potential sweeps down the axon into the axon terminals,
special calcium ion gates in the terminals open suddenly, causing Ca^{++}
to enter the terminals. The calcium spike causes membrane-lined vesicles containing specialized chemicals known as neurotransmitters to fuse
with the axon terminus (the presynaptic membrane). As these synaptic
vesicles fuse with the presynaptic membrane they burst much like a soap
bubble coming into contact with a surface. The contents of the vesicles
are thus released into the synaptic cleft—the small gap separating the
axonal tip from the postsynaptic membrane on the adjacent neuron. The
neurotransmitters activate specific receptors on the postsynaptic membrane,
causing ionic gates to open. Thus the action potential causes neurotransmitters to activate receptors on the postsynaptic membrane, giving
rise to graded potentials, which can be either excitatory or inhibitory
depending upon the specific ionic gates opening in response. Action
potentials are produced by changes in the electrical charge distribution
of the neural membrane; they are thus voltage-gated. Graded potentials,
on the other hand, are produced by the action of specific chemical
neurotransmitters at postsynaptic receptors; they are thus chemically-gated.

One of the most abundant neurotransmitters is acetylcholine, synthesized from a vitamin, choline, by attaching an acetyl group in a reaction
facilitated by the enzyme choline acetyltransferase. The enzyme and the
acetyl group are synthesized in the cell body of the neuron and transported to the axon terminal by axoplasmic flow. Choline is carried across
the terminal membrane from the blood by a carrier protein. Like other
neurotransmitters, acetylcholine is degraded by enzymes, in this case
acetylcholine esterase, and it is packaged into synaptic vesicles to prevent degradation and to store it for release when needed. There are some
10,000 molecules of acetylcholine in each synaptic vesicle and two acetylcholine molecules are required to activate one cholinergic receptor.
When this happens, the receptor protein undergoes a stereochemical
change which opens the ion channel. Once the receptors are activated in
response to a stimulus, the remaining acetylcholine molecules must be

broken down or cleared from the synapse to prevent uncontrolled, machinegunlike firing—this would precipitate a seizure in short order. This breakdown and clearance is accomplished by acetylcholine esterase and by presynaptic reuptake of those acetylcholine molecules not degraded by the enzyme.

The action of acetylcholine is an example of a one-messenger system of synaptic transmission. In this case the messenger is acetylcholine itself, and the receptors are activated directly and the associated ionic gates are opened. Other major neurotransmitters, including the monoamines and oligopeptide transmitters, are generally operated by means of a two-messenger system. In this type of action, the neurotransmitter serves as the first messenger; it operates the receptor site. The receptor is closely associated with an enzyme, adenylate cyclase, which is activated by the receptor. The activated adenylate cyclase splits two phosphate groups from ATP, converting it into a very active molecule, cyclic AMP. Cyclic AMP in turn activates a kinase (another enzyme) which takes the two phosphates cleaved from the ATP and phosphorylates a membrane protein which functions as an ionic gate. The ionic gate absorbs the energy in the phosphate groups and changes stereochemically to permit ionic influx. In this system, cAMP acts as the second messenger. Cyclic AMP continues to activate protein kinases until it is deactivated by cyclic nucleotide phosphodiesterase. Thus a small number of neurotransmitter molecules can indirectly produce a much larger number of activated kinase molecules, resulting in a greatly amplified neuronal response relative to the limited number of receptor sites that are occupied.

The three major monoamine neurotransmitters are dopamine, norepinephrine, and serotonin (5-hydroxyindoletryptamine or 5-HT). These are synthesized in the axon terminal from amino acid precursors transported into the terminals from the blood by carrier proteins. Tyrosine is the precursor for dopamine and dopamine is the precursor for norepinephrine. Tryptophan is the precursor for 5-HT. The monoamine transmitters are cleared from the synapse after their release by presynaptic reuptake, as in the case of acetylcholine, and by chemical degradation by the enzymes, monoamine oxidase (MAO) and catechol-O-methyl transferase (COMT) or by COMT's analogue, 5-hydroxyindole-O-methyltransferase (5-HIOMT), in the case of serotonin. These enzymes operate alternately on each molecule of monoamine transmitter and convert it into its aldehyde intermediate. The aldehyde intermediate is then oxidized by aldehyde dehydrogenase into its organic acid or reduced by alcohol deyhdrogenase into its respective alcohol (see Light 1985 for a discussion of alcohol and aldehyde chemistry).

In addition to the monoamines, a number of amino acids and short-length peptide sequences also act as central neurotransmitters. The amino acids glutamate and aspartate act as excitatory transmitters whereas glycine and GABA are strong inhibitory substances. Among the peptide chains are the widely publicized endogenous opiates: the endorphins and enkephalins which bind to the same receptors in the CNS as do opiate derivatives such as morphine, heroin and codeine. The enkephalins are released in response to psychic and/or physical pain and stress. They bind to receptor sites on larger axons, preventing the latter from releasing their own neurotransmitters and thus breaking the circuit. Enkephalins are highly concentrated in certain parts of the spinal cord and in the limbic system and hypothalamus in the brain. In the spinal cord they prevent pain-bearing neurons from releasing substance P, known to be involved in the mediation of physical pain. In the limbic system they reduce the stress resulting from physical or psychological pain so that it is no longer perceived as a negative experience.

Neuroendocrine transducers constitute a special type of neurotransmission. These neurons terminate in bulbous axonal endings instead of typical terminal buttons, and they contain both neurotransmitter vesicles and neurosecretory vesicles, the latter containing special neurohormones. Hormones are substances which are released into the blood for action on target cells at a distance from the point of their release. The bulbous endings of neuroendocrine transducers are in contact with blood capillaries, forming a neurohaemal organ. Action potentials sweeping into the bulbous axonal ending elicit the release of the neurotransmitter substances into the bulbous axonal ending itself, causing the neurosecretory vesicles to fuse with the presynaptic membrane and release their neurohormones into the blood stream. These neuroendocrine transducers are very abundant in the hypothalamus of the brain and they release hormones that exert specific actions on the anterior lobe of the pituitary gland or upon other tissues in the body. Hypophysiotropic neurohormones stimulate the anterior pituitary to release such hormones as thyroid-stimulating hormone, growth hormone (somatotropin), adrenocorticotropic hormone, and the reproductive hormones like follicle-stimulating hormone and luteinizing hormone. Examples of hormones released by the hypothalamus for action at distant target tissues include vasopressin (antidiuretic hormone), which permits water retention by the kidneys, and oxytocin, which acts upon the uterus and mammary glands during labor and lactation, respectively.

The nervous system is organized into two major categories: (1) the central nervous system or CNS which includes the brain and its derivatives and the spinal cord, and (2) the peripheral nervous system consisting of the nerve pathways running from the base of the brain and the spinal cord out to the peripheral regions of the body where they receive a variety of signals and deliver commands from the CNS. Aggregates of nerve cell bodies within the CNS are termed nuclei; such aggregates in the peripheral nervous system are called ganglia.

The peripheral nervous system is divided into the somatic nervous system and the autonomic nervous system. The somatic nervous system includes spinal pathways receiving sensory input from outlying receptor organs and innervating motor pathways which exercise voluntary control over the skeletal muscles. The somatic nervous system also includes a wide variety of reflex arcs, the basic functional unit of the nervous system; these permit rapid action at the spinal level to avoid dangerous situations such as a hot stove long before the individual becomes consciously aware that he or she has been burned. Although the somatic nervous system is involved in those operations under conscious, voluntary control, reflex arcs themselves are quite involuntary.

The autonomic nervous system innervates the viscera and smooth ("involuntary") muscles which move those organs. Autonomic pathways are normally not under voluntary control, although many mystics, *yogis* and Zen-men have trained themselves to this ability. The autonomic nervous system is divided into two components: (1) the sympathetic system and (2) the parasympathetic system. Sympathetic nerves innervate the viscera and especially the adrenal medullae and generally prepare the body for extreme emergencies in the fight or flight response. They cause the adrenals to pour out norepinephrine and epinephrine, which in turn stimulate the heart into accelerated activity, increase peripheral vasoconstriction and elevate blood pressure. They stimulate glycogen release by the liver and lower blood insulin levels, thus maintaining blood glucose concentrations. The pituitary is also stimulated into releasing adrenocorticotropic hormone, which cause the adrenal cortices to release hydrocortisone (cortisol) which counters some of the effects of epinephrine upon blood glucose levels. Both epinephrine and cortisol mobilize peripheral free fatty acids and enhance beta-oxidation for the quick production of energy.

The parasympathetic system acts to restore normal physiological balance after the emergency has been survived. Unlike the sympathetic system, which is spinal in origin, the parasympathetic system is cranial and sacral. The sympathetic system releases norepinephrine at the postganglionic synapses, whereas the parasympathetic system is entirely cholinergic. All cholinergic receptors throughout the somatic and sympathetic systems and most of the parasympathetic system are nicotinic; however, the postganglionic parasympathetic receptors are muscarinic. Nicotinic cholinergic receptors are activated by acetylcholine in a one-messenger system; muscarinic receptors are two-messenger systems involving both acetylcholine and cyclic GMP (cyclic guanosine monophosphate). Muscarinic receptors are very abundant in the cortex of the brain as well as in the mid- and lower-brain, but nicotinic receptors also occur in these places.

The primitive brain (both evolutionarily and embryologically speaking) is a tube which forms a series of swollen chambers connected by constrictions. These swellings divide the primitive brain into the following divisions: (1) the forebrain or telencephalon, including the two cerebral hemispheres (first two ventricles), and the diencephalon (third brain ventricle); (2) the midbrain or mesencephalon; and (3) the hindbrain or rhombencephalon. The two cerebral hemispheres of the telencephalon are also composed of the following evolutionary and embryogenic grades of organization: the paleocortex or "ancient brain," the archicortex or "old brain," and the neocortex or "new brain." The paleocortex gives rise in the higher mammals to the basal ganglia of the limbic system. The archicortex is destined to form the hippocampus, and the neocortex forms the complex and highly advanced cerebral cortex where advanced intelligence and information processing occur in the higher mammals, including man.

As the brain develops, the two cerebral hemispheres expand laterally and rearwards and they come to sit over the lower portions of the brain like a mushroom on its stem. The neocortex is the uppermost portion and it is the seat of highest mental activity and integration. The limbic system is a series of large ganglia underlying the neocrotex, but surrounding lower forebrain. It is the seat where emotional experience occurs. The limbic system contains three large, paired ganglia or nuclei: the caudate nucleus, putamen and globus pallidus; the latter two collectively comprise the corpus striatum. The corpus striatum acts in concert with the cerebellum to control motor coordination. Dopamine-releasing neurons from a center in the brainstem known as the substantia nigra exert an inhibitory control over the striatum and the adjacent thalamus. If too many of these cells die off, the resulting inhibitory release upon the striatum produces the uncontrolled jerking movements seen in Parkinson's syndrome.

The third ventricle is surrounded by the diencephalon, of which the two lateral walls constitute the thalamus and the floor comprises the hypothalamus. The thalamus is the major relay station of the brain, routing incoming signals to the appropriate areas of the cortex for processing and sending commands to the proper lower nervous pathways. A deep pit in the floor of the hypothalamus is called the infundibulum and its anterior wall forms the posterior lobe of the pituitary gland (neurohypophysis); during embryogenesis a pouch forms in the roof of the pharynx which breaks off and migrates to fuse with the neurohypophysis, forming the anterior lobe of the pituitary (adenohypophysis). Two ventral, breastlike swellings projecting downwards from the posterior surface of the hypothalamus form the mammillary bodies. These are involved in the mediation of aggression and rage, and together with the paired hippocampi, are involved in learning and short-term memory. The hypothalamus is the site where emotions are expressed, and it is involved in the regulation of hunger, thirst and sexual activity. The optic nerves and retinae of the eyes are formed from lateral outgrowths of the diencephalon and they are an integral part of the brain itself.

The dorsal portion of the anterior part of the hindbrain develops into the cerebellum, which together with the striatum and thalamus is involved in motor coordination. Most of the brain provides a strong defense against the introduction of foreign molecules known as the blood-brain barrier. The dense packing of myelinated fibers and 100 billion or so supporting cells of the brain effectively prevent the diffusion of most substances into the neurons of the brain, thus preserving a fairly constant internal environment. Lying dorsally between the telencephalon and diencephalon and just posterior to the cerebellum, however, are two richly vascularized, thin and pleated sheets of tissue called the choroid plexi. These blood-rich regions provide ready access to the brain for such small molecules as glucose, oxygen, amino acids and psychotropic drugs of all kinds. Lying posterior to the hypothalamus and ventral and posterior to the cerebellum of the primitive brain is the hindbrain, where basic physiological functions such as heartbeat and breathing are regulated.

The brain is thus arranged into a series of concentric shells in descending order of evolutionary and developmental complexity and advancement. The higher neocortex regulates and inhibits the underlying limbic system. It thus screens and edits emotional experience to the appropriateness of the circumstances in which the individual finds himself. The limbic system in turn exerts control over the diencephalic centers, including the thalamus and hypothalamus. And the hypothalamus controls the underlying midbrain and brainstem.

The reticular formation is a complex network of interconnected neurons lying within the brainstem. Major ascending fibers radiate upward from the reticular formation to all parts of the cerebral cortex. This system is known as the reticular activating system or R.A.S. It is in a constant state of spontaneous activity, and it continually maintains a state of cortical arousal and mental alertness. The thalamus is also involved in the system and mediates selective attention so that an individual can focus upon a single situation or subject. The thalamus is also the site where extraneous and nonsignificant stimuli are screened from consciousness, thus providing for accommodation. Without this capacity for accommodation, we would be driven quite mad from the continual bombardment of stimuli from the environment.

The sleep-wake cycle is regulated by two neuronal centers in the hindbrain: the serotonin-releasing neurons of the raphe nuclei and the adrenergic neurons of the locus coeruleus. The raphe nuclei inhibit the R.A.S. and produce unconsciousness. At regular intervals the raphe nuclei back off, releasing part of their inhibition upon the R.A.S. Simultaneously, signals from the locus coeruleus to descending pathways cause all bodily movements to cease. At the same time, the locus coeruleus prompts the R.A.S. into moderate arousal. This produces rapid-eye movements and the semi-conscious state we know as dreaming. Because signals from the cortex can produce arousal in the R.A.S., situational or neurotic conflict counters the effects of the raphe nuclei and results in insomnia. Psychological depression and anxiety resulting from both neurotic tension and specific biochemical imbalances of central neurotransmitters involving both serotonin and norepinephrine, produce severe and chronic insomnia in millions of individuals. This results in the use and abuse of prescription and over-the-counter sleep-inducing drugs on a huge scale.

Tryptophan is a poor competitor for the carrier proteins that transport amino acids inside cells. A high-carbohydrate meal just before bedtime results in insulin release, and this results in the clearance of all amino acids from the blood except for tryptophan. Tryptophan is thus left with few competitors for the carrier-protein system, it is readily carried into axonal endings and converted into serotonin, and tends to counter insomnia. Avoidance of high-protein meals also reduce the blood levels of amino acids. Milk has a high tryptophan content and it is also effective in countering insomnia. Rage and aggression also involve interplay between serotonin and norepinephrine, and serotonin and tryptophan tend to inhibit rage responses, although cholinergic pathways are also involved.

BIOLOGY, PSYCHIATRY, DRUGS, AND THE ACTIONS OF ALCOHOL

With the foregoing brief, if rather intensive, overview of neurology behind us we are now ready to discuss the biochemical dynamics underlying certain psychiatric disorders, the various chemotherapies used to treat these disorders, and why they work as they do. The psychodynamic and sociological factors underlying such psychiatric processes are treated in the third volume in this series (Light, in press, Volume 3), where they will be integrated with the biochemical parameters presented here. This section will conclude with a detailed treatment of the pharmacological actions of alcohol upon the human nervous system. The interaction of alcohol and other psychotropic drugs, including caffeine and tobacco, are treated in Volume 4 of this series.

DEPRESSION, MEDICINE, AND ALCOHOL

It has already been stated that depression is closely associated with deficits in the levels and/or activity of norepinephrine and serotonin. This is now clearly established and is accepted by the great majority of psychiatrists and other physicians. Some psychologists, however, many of whom have little training in the medical aspects of psychiatric disturbances, and who appear to be threatened by medical models, insist that no such biological factors play any role in the development of mental illness. They are in the minority, nevertheless, and the overwhelming burden of evidence supports the medical models pertaining to these disorders.

Until quite recently the conventional wisdom was that depression fell into two quite distinct and neat categories: *endogenous* or *primary depression* and *exogenous* or *secondary*[30] *depression.* Endogenous depression

---

[30]Exogenous or secondary depression is also frequently called *reactive* or *neurotic depression.* The details of these disorders are treated in detail in Volume 3 of this series.

exhibits clear genetic inheritance patterns and is also genetically associated with primary alcoholism. Endogenous depression is the direct
result of neurotransmitter deficiencies—specifically of serotonin and
norepinephrine—and it is generally treated with medications which
correct those deficiencies. Reactive depression, by contrast, has traditionally been considered to be psychogenically caused and the preferred
treatment has been typically intensive individual psychoanalytic psychotherapy[31] to resolve the emotional conflicts underlying the disorder.
Antidepressant medications were not generally considered to be of much
benefit in alleviating reactive depression because it was thought not to
involve biochemical imbalances in the brain. Some short-term chemotherapy with anti-anxiety benzodiazepenes such as chlordiazepoxide
(Librium®) and diazepam (Valium®) are often used in such cases, however,
to help the patient through periods of extreme anxiety or tension and to
alleviate depression-associated insomnia.

More recently, however, a growing number of physicians—particularly
family and general practice physicians—are successfully employing tricyclic and the closely related tetracyclic antidepressant medications with
patients presenting with so-called "neurotic" depression. These agents
frequently greatly improve or totally eliminate these depressions after
the initial "incubation" period of from one to three weeks has passed.[32]
Many psychiatrists still insist that such medications cannot work in the
case of "psychogenically" caused depression, but the plain fact is that
most patients treated in this manner respond extremely well to such
management. Although I will explore this subject in more detail further
on in this book, suffice it for the moment to say that endogenous and
reactive depression appear to represent two extremes of a continuum
and that there appears to be a genetic factor involved in all cases of
clinical depression involving serotonin and/or norepinephrine deficiencies
in the brain. Many of the features formerly thought to distinguish the

---

[31]Psychoanalytic psychotherapy refers to the traditional, Freudian psychoanalytic approach in which the
therapist and patient jointly explore the unresolved narcissistic and oedipal conflicts thought to underlie
maladaptive and inappropriate adult behavior. Such an approach is very similar to classical psychoanalysis,
but it is much less intense and of shorter duration. Instead of spending 50 minutes five days a week on the
analyst's couch for ten years or so, the patient sees the therapist once or twice a week for one to four or five
years, depending upon the patient's progress and the goals set. Furthermore, the patient usually does not
lie on a couch but sits facing the therapist.

[32]For reasons that are totally obscure, the tricyclic antidepressants require up to 3 to 4 weeks before they
become effective. The related tetracyclics such as Maprotiline (Ludiomil®) are usually effective within one
week.

two types (such as *early* versus *terminal insomnia* and diurnal cyclic mood swings as contrasted with invariant dysphoria throughout the day) are commonly seen to blend into each other and the diagnosis itself may change over the course of the disorder. This last point is, by the way, a very critical one! Psychiatric disorders commonly evolve and change over their course, and what begins as one often rather confused diagnostic entity may very well wind up being clearly diagnosed as something quite different as the disorder "matures" into a more classical symptomatic portrait. It is not uncommon for a patient long classified as having, say, *schizoaffective schizophrenia* which responds only poorly to phenothiazine therapy to finally be diagnosed as having a manic disorder, and very effectively treated with lithium salts.

Depressions are either *unipolar* or *bipolar.* Unipolar depressions involve one or more episodes of depression only, and they may be *chronic* or *recurrent.* Chronic depressions tend to be more or less lifelong and unremitting, and they do not usually respond to changing, more favorable life circumstances. Recurrent depressions are often very severe and totally disabling and they tend to occur repeatedly with intervening periods of clarity and good social and psychological functioning during which the patient exhibits a cheerful and out-going, pleasant affect. These depressive episodes are typically self-limiting and they tend to terminate sponteneously, usually within 6 months or a year regardless of treatment. Bipolar depression involves at least one *manic* or *hypomanic* episode alternating with one or more depressive phases.[33]Mania is the exact opposite of depression and it appears to be at least partly caused by excessive brain levels of norepinephrine—precisely the reverse of the neurotransmitter imbalance associated with depression. Both severe mania and depression are very dangerous states; the depressive is always an obvious suicide risk and manic patients may violently resist any attempt to interfere with or alter their activity and homicides are not unknown. Bipolar swings between mania and depression have given rise to the term *manic-depressive disorder* commonly applied to this disorder. Persons who exhibit cyclic swings between cheerfulness and accelerated

---

[33]Very briefly, mania or its less severe manifestation, *hypomania,* is characterized by extreme psychomotor acceleration and an unrealistic optimism about actual and projected future achievements which are not justified by the circumstances. The extreme cheerfulness seen in some manic patients becomes extreme irritability, anger and impatience in others. Manics often exhibit *clang associations* where words are connected by their sounds rather than their meaning. Double and triple entendres, multiple puns and fanciful *flights of ideas* are also commonly seen. Clang associations are also typical of certain cases of schizophrenia and they often confuse the diagnosis.

thinking and activity on the one hand and depression and retarded activity and thinking (or its equivalent, agitation and irritability) on the other, but who do not exhibit a severe enough pathology to warrant the diagnosis of manic-depressive disorder, are said to have a *cyclothymic personality. Depressive spectrum disorder* refers to depression in an individual coming from a family in which alcoholism and/or sociopathy is also present in one or more members. In such families, females are more commonly depressed and males are more likely to exhibit alcoholism, sociopathy, or both.

Finally, depression may be either *retarded* or *agitated.* Retarded depression is more common and it is characterized by often extremely inhibited physical, mental and emotional activity. The patient may require many minutes before answering a simple question and present a posture, facial features, and affect signaling profound apathy, helplessness and a sense of utter despair and hopelessness. Quite obviously, this is a very extreme example and the entire spectrum from near normal functioning and affect to that just described may occur. Retarded depression may be associated primarily with deficits of norepinephrine. Agitated depression typically exhibits much agitation, irritibility often with explosive outbursts of temper, pacing and wringing of hands, and usually very severe insomnia (typically early insomnia; see footnote 39). This type of depression may involve brain deficits of both norepinephrine and serotonin, and much of the irritability, anger and rage reactions exhibited may involve inadequate inhibition by serotonin on the amygdaloid centers controlling the expression of hypothalamic rage.

Serotonin inhibits the amygdaloid nuclei, a part of the limbic system closely involved with the conscious experience of emotion (see figures 19 and 20). A serotonin deficit releases that inhibition and is equivalent to the stimulation of those nuclei. The immediate consequences are anxiety and depression—symptoms of psychic stress. Stimulation of the amygdala causes enhanced production of hydrocortisol (see figure 14). In addition to the massive metabolic disruption this causes, often leading to effective hypoglycemia and severe emotional stress which further compounds the initial anxiety and depression, cortisol stimulates the release of *tryptophan pyrrolase* in the liver, an enzyme which enhances the degradation of tryptophan and deprives the brain of the precursor amino acid required to synthesize 5-hydroxytryptamine (serotonin). The original deficiency of serotonin results in the effective stimulation of the amygdala, which in turn stimulates the release of hydrocortisol by the adrenal cortices, stimulating the production of tryptophan pyrrolase within the liver, which enhances the breakdown of tryptophan and thus inhibits still further the synthesis of serotonin. Thus, a vicious, positively reinforced spiral of events occurs leading to more severe, escalating psychological disturbances accompanied by physiological changes which feed back into the original imbalance. It is noteworthy that chronic alcohol ingestion by laboratory animals results in decreased activity of tryptophan pyrrolase in the brain (Noble & Tewari 1978). However, acute ethanol administration increases hepatic trypotphan pyrrolase activity (Shaw & Lieber 1979).

Finally, decreased availability of serotonin and the consequent inhibitory release of the reticular activating system causes hyperactivity of the R.A.S. leading to enhanced cortical activity and anxiety, agitation and insomnia. Although by no means demonstrated, this may interfere with the mechanisms within the reticular formation involved in selective attention, accommodation, and psychological repression, that is in filtering out extraeneous and unwanted stimuli.

As we have seen, the reticular activating system constitutes an arousing mechanism; when stimulated it enhances consciousness and increases alertness, and when inhibited these two functions are likewise diminished. Stimuli from the environment are sent to the thalamus whence they are evaluated and sent on to the appropriate cortical centers. They are also sent directly to the cerebral cortex via direct pathways (figure 21A). In addition, such stimuli enter the reverberating network of the reticular formation where they lose their specificity and are amplified many times, causing general arousing signals to go out along the ascending fibers of the R.A.S. to the neocortex. Because of the diffuseness of the R.A.S., quite different sensory signals generate equal activation and consciousness arousal. The cerebral cortex integrates both the direct, specific sensory messages and the general arousal signals and sends impulses back to the R.A.S. which either enhance or reduce its activity.

The R.A.S. is involved in both selective attention (which is under cortical and thalamic control) and sensory habituation. Lesions or drugs which inhibit neuronal activity in the reticular formation prevent the development of normal habituation in experimental animals. Furthermore, previously habituated animals are permanently released from the habituation (Kaplan & Sadock, 1980). Left to its own devices the R.A.S. remains in a state of constant, spontaneous arousal, resulting in increased consciousness and enhanced alertness of the organism. Paradoxically, however, R.A.S. activity also exerts an inhibitory action upon those functions involved in the focusing of selective attention and sensory habituation. The R.A.S. is more active (and thus selectively inhibits more) under conditions of routine sensory input.

Stimulation of the R.A.S. thus has both excitatory and inhibitory effects. This confusing situation can perhaps be partly accounted for by the existence of central feedback inhibition loops. The firing of a seretonin-releasing neuron (1) excites the postsynaptic, serotoninoceptive neuron (2), which in turn stimulates neurons (3 *et seq.*) further along in the pathway or network. However, a collateral fiber from neuron (2) excites one or more inhibitory neurons (4), which then inhibit the firing of the original neuron (1). Thus:

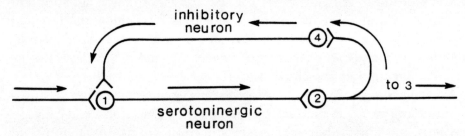

R.A.S. dysfunction has been suggested as a precipitating factor in a number of psychiatric syndromes. *Childhood hyperkinesis* is characterized by overactivity, attention deficit disorder and distractibility, irritability, impulsiveness, low frustration tolerance, and poor school performance. The fact that amphetamine therapy, which enhances the activity of dopamine receptors in the thalamus and corpus striatum and which control reticular activity, is so effective in alleviating this disorder suggests that dysfunction of the reticular formation may be involved. *Narcolepsy* begins in youth or early adulthood. It is characterized, among other things, by sudden and irresistible desire for sleep. There may also be minor to profound, transient loss of body muscle tone, a state termed *cataplexy;* there may even be total flaccid paralysis while entering or emerging from sleep. Lesions of the reticular formation have been demonstrated in these patients, and large doses of amphetamines are beneficial. Interestingly, cataplexy responds to imipramine, one of the tricyclic antidepressants! The global cognitive disorganization and disintergration of the rational association of emotions and thoughts within a coherent context so evident in schizophrenic decompensation is also thought to be the result of R.A.S. hyperarousal. An excess of dopamine or at least of dopamine receptors in the thalamus is known to be a major biochemical correlative of schizophrenia. The phenothiazine drugs used in the treatment of these disorders act to block dopamine receptors and thus reduce the effects of that neurotransmitter within the thalamus. Large doses of amphetamines produce a toxic psychosis which is often very hard to distinguish clinically from paranoid schizophrenia. Amphetamines enhance the effects of dopamine within the thalamus and corpus striatum, and the phenothiazines are effective antagonists to the amphetamines. The administration of chlorpromazine (Thorazine®, one of the first pheothiazines employed) eliminates the effects of electrical stimulation of the reticular formation in laboratory rats (Kaplan & Sadock 1980).

The exact balance between excitation and inhibition resulting from neurotransmitter imbalances, lesions, and hyper- or hypoactivity of the various components of the reticular formation, thalamus, and ascending reticular pathways cannot, of course, really be predicted. A serotonin deficit like that seen in many cases of depression has multiple and often contradictory effects. On the one hand, reduced serotonin levels in the brain release the inhibition the raphe nuclei exert upon the R.A.S. resulting in hyperarousal of that system. This can cause agitation, restlessness and severe insomnia. On the other hand, such a deficiency reduces the feedback inhibition to the serotoninergic neurons, indirectly increasing their level of activity. This increased activity may then: (1) elevate the turnover rate for serotonin, further depleting that substance, and (2) cause enhanced inhibition and/or excitation of various portions of the R.A.S. The poor filtering (repressive) competence of the selective attention and habituation mechanisms seen in many depressed alcoholics may very well at least partly result from reticular dysfunction. This idea has been suggested by several investigators and I believe it has much merit.

Persons with high tonic arousal associated with R.A.S. hyperactivity exhibit a marked decrease of such arousal after ethanol administration during which they experience pleasure. Drugs, such as alcohol and the barbiturates, which exert a generalized fluidizing effect upon neural membranes (see below) as contrasted with those like the benzodiazepenes which operate primarily at specific receptor sites, tend to affect multisynaptic neural networks much more profoundly than they do simpler synaptic pathways.[34] Thus, the cerebral cortex with its cognitive and inhibitory functions and the R.A.S. with its arousal, selective attention, habituation, and screening mechanisms are the first systems to be affected by ethanol, and they are affected to a much greater extent than are most other CNS systems.

Ethanol in low doses facilitates neural activity by inhibiting the sodium-potassium pump, (see also below, page 95), whereas in higher doses it suppresses neural transmission by distorting membrane architecture and rendering the ionic gates effectively inoperable (figure 23). The slight facilitation of neural activity occurring with small amounts of ethanol probably partly contributes to the "conviviality" induced by social drinking. This results from the slightly increased arousal of the R.A.S. which simultaneously elevates overall arousal and alertness and enhances the inhibitory effects of the R.A.S. upon the selective attention and screening mechanisms of the thalamic portion of the recticular activating system. In the case of impaired diencephalic (thalamic) screening processes which I believe exist in many alcoholics, this enhanced R.A.S. inhibition permits the individual to finally relegate the constant bombardment of extraneous and unwanted stimuli, thoughts and emotions to the pre-conscious portions of the mind and to attend more easily and with less distraction to the situations at hand (the social or sexual interaction) without the anxieties generated by superego failure. Initial stimulation of the R.A.S. increases its inhibitory as well as its arousal actions within the CNS, and anxiety and tension resulting from pre- and unconscious material intruding constantly into conscious awareness is accordingly diminished.

With increased alcohol intake, the initial slight stimulatory effect upon neural membranes is quickly replaced by a much stronger depressant action. The influx of sodium ions required to depolarize or reverse the membrane potential necessary to generating an nervous impulse is progressively blocked as more alcohol is consumed. This depressant action is also more pronounced within the reverberating and self-propagating neuronal networks of the cerebral cortex, the reticular formation, and to a lesser extent, the motor coordination centers of the cerebellum. Both cognitive and emotional functions are among the first

---

[34]Barbiturates also act at specific receptor sites closely associated, like the benzodiazepine receptors, with GABA-receptors. Because of their global effects on reverberating circuits, however, barbiturate-induced coma is much more profound than that produced by benzodiazepines.

to be affected. As the neocortex becomes progressively depressed, its inhibitory actions upon the limbic system and R.A.S. are also lifted. This inhibitory release allows emotions and affective states normally under cortical control to bubble over into consciousness and overt behavior. With increasing intoxication the individual may exhibit increasingly less inhibited behavior, becoming voluble, loquacious, and very much the unself-conscious *bon vivant* of the social gathering. This superficial hyperarousal is appropriately enough known as paradoxical excitement because it is due primarily to the release of cortical inhibition. At the same time that inhibitions upon the R.A.S. are being lifted because of cortical depression, the spontaneous activity of the activating system is also being severely depressed by the drug. The actual point where these two conflicting activity curves intersect is unclear, but it seems certain that the general depressant effect of ethanol upon the R.A.S. greatly overrides any increase in activity resulting from inhibitory release (see also figure 24). This effect becomes progressively greater as drinking continues. Moreover, as cortical disinhibition allows ever deeper levels of emotional material to surge into "consciousness," the corresponding decrease in cognitive awareness resulting from neocortical depression more than compensates for any "censorship-failure anxiety" that might otherwise occur. For alcoholics, the bottom line is always that alcohol permits a blessed escape from the constant state of anxiety and tension resulting from the failure of both physiological and psychological repressive mechanisms.[35]

Electroencephalographic (EEG) profiles are the result of complex interactions at several different levels of the brain. EEG waves, and in particular alpha-waves, are produced by the cerebral cortex and coordinated by a group of interdependent "pacemakers" located in the thalamus. These thalamic pacemakers are, in turn, modulated by lower brain input—particularly from the reticular activating system. A high level of R.A.S. arousal results in a desynchronized EEG pattern and poor alpha-activity in the resting state. A strong alpha-rhythm is associated with emotional stability, resistance to stress, and a general feeling of serenity and well-being. A variety of meditation and bio-feedback techniques are known to enhance alpha-activity as well as enkephalin release, thus

---

[35]It must be noted here that the decompensation of repressive functions in alcoholics is due to a physiological deficit as well as being the direct result of the psychological consequences of narcissistic trauma and entitlement loss, from which springs lowered self-esteem coupled with the expectation of rejection, and obsessive-compulsive traits associated with loss of power.

promoting a positive affect. EEG patterns are almost completely genetically determined, as has been determined by concordance studies on
monozygotic (identical) and dizygotic (fraternal) twin pairs.

The EEG response to ethanol intake varies at least partly as a function
of the individual's typical resting pattern. Those with a strong and stable
resting alpha-rhythm show relatively little EEG change in response to an
ethanol challenge. However, those persons with a poor resting alpha-
rhythm respond strongly to an alcohol challenge by producing a much
stronger and more stable alpha-pattern than existed prior to the challenge.
Furthermore, the change in EEG pattern produced by ethanol persists
long after most of the drug has been cleared from the body. These
individual differences in EEG pattern produced by ethanol are under
strong genetic determination.

EEG studies have consistently shown that alcoholics tend to have a
poorly developed alpha-rhythm, and in fact, the alpha-pattern exhibited
by this group is similar to that seen in individuals who react to ethanol
by developing a strong, and long-lasting alpha-pattern. In view of the
close association between strong alpha-activity and a peaceful relaxed
state on the one hand, and of high tonic arousal, stress and dysphoria
with poor alpha-activity on the other, the implication that susceptible
individuals might be prone to self-medicate with ethanol seems obvious.
This notion is certainly in agreement with the observations that alcoholics and prealcoholics respond in a unique way to ethanol—alcohol does
something very special to this population that is simply not experienced
by nonalcoholic persons. The state of chronic high tonic arousal and
dysphoria experienced by alcoholically predisposed individuals is readily alleviated by beverage alcohol; the person feels better and is able to
operate more fluently in interpersonal relationships (both at home and
on the job). This positive reinforcement is conducive to still more reliance upon alcohol, and the alcoholic downward spiral is underway.

Recent studies (Pollock *et al.* 1983; Curran 1983) have shown that the
distinctive pattern of brain waves exhibited by alcoholics are also seen in
their male offspring. Many of the sons of alcoholic probands exhibit the
same brain wave deficits as severe alcoholics *even though these sons had no
prior exposure to alcohol!* Nor had the mothers of these boys drunk during
pregnancy. When given alcohol for the first time in an experimental
setting, The EEG's of these subjects were identical to the responses of
chronic alcoholics to an ethanol challenge. None of the age-matched
controls (sons of nonalcoholic parents) exhibited any of these abnormal

responses. These aberrant brain-wave patterns in chronic alcoholics were previously thought to result from alcohol-induced brain damage, but their existence in the sons of alcoholics prior to any ethanol insult strongly suggests that they are genetically predetermined. These pre-alcoholic, poorly developed alpha-waves are known to correlate with stress, anxiety and dysphoria (see above), which respond to ethanol by much greater decreases in fast alpha-activity and increases in slow alpha-activity relative to normal controls. This may very well reflect the increased psychic tension and exaggerated relief obtained from alcohol intake seen in alcoholics. As the author states (Curran 1983): "For those with a genetic predisposition to alcoholism, alcohol may have a positive reinforcing effect by slowing brain activity. Thirty-nine percent of the biological sons of alcoholic fathers showed these aberrant brain waves, which were generated primarily in the hippocampus and limbic system. This figure closely approximates the reports of other investigators that 30–40% of the sons of alcoholic fathers will themselves also become alcoholic."

Depression, as I have said, is known to involve deficits in both serotonin and norepinephrine. This appears to be the case regardless of whether the depression is primarily endogenous (primary) or reactive (secondary). Serotonin is primarily an inhibitory transmitter, particularly in the reticular activating system. However, it also has excitatory functions especially within certain parts of the limbic system. Both serotonin and norepinephrine occur most abundantly in the phylogenetically older regions of the brain, although norepinephrine is also found peripherally in the sympathetic postganglionic fibers as we have seen. Within the CNS, norepinephrine is concentrated mainly in the hypothalamus, hippocampus, cerebral cortex, reticular formation and the spinal cord, and the cerebellum. The relative activities of these two neurotransmitters appear to be at least partly responsible for the clinical differences exhibited by the range of depressed patients. Retarded patients are likely to suffer primarily from a norepinephrine deficit, whereas norepinephrine coupled with serotonin deficiency appears to be involved in the case of agitated and angry depressed patients. *Melatonin* is another indoleamine which is synthesized from serotonin in two steps within the pineal gland by the enzymes *alkylamine N-acetyltransferase* and *N-acetylserotonin O-methyltransferase*. Melatonin, which is highly concentrated in the pineal body, is an important chemical agent in the regulation of *circadian rhythms*—the diurnal variations of a number of physiological functions governed by our innate biological clocks. Melatonin levels and N-acetyltransferase activity are normally highest at night. A deficit in the precursor, serotonin, directly affects the levels of pineal melatonin, and the ensuing nocturnal deficit of melatonin may play an added role in depressive insomnia. Chlorpromazine is sometimes used in the treatment of agitated depression characterized by severe insomnia. In addition to its usual anti-psychotic activity[36] it also inhibits the metabolism of melatonin, resulting in the increased retention and thus effective enhanced levels and activity of that substance. This very likely accounts for its efficacy in such cases of depression.

Abnormal cortisol (hydrocortisone) release profiles have been linked to both childhood and adult depression (Cytryn & McKnew 1980). Corticotrophin or adrenocorticotrophic hormone (ACTH) is released from the adenohypophysis in response to corticotrophin-releasing hormone (C–RH) from the median eminence of the hypothalamus (see above, figures 12 and 14). ACTH stimulates the cortex of the adrenal glands to release both cortisol and mineralcorticoids. ACTH, and thus also cortisol release, is inhibited by a negative feedback mechanism operating upon a norepinephrine-mediated pathway within the hypothalamus. As cortisol is released it acts upon specific norepinephrine-releasing neurons which synapse with C–RH releasing neuroendocrine transducers within the arcuate and tuberal nuclei of the median eminence (figure 14).

The administration of a synthetic glucocorticoid, *dexamethasone*, causes a negative feedback suppression of endogenous corticotrophin in normal persons via these noradrenergic neurons, thus inhibiting C–RH release by the neuroendocrine transducers. Depressed patients typically show an abnormal response to the *dexamethasone suppression test:* because of a central norepinephrine deficit, this negative feedback pathway is interrupted and there is no ensuing depression of ACTH or cortisol following dexamethasone administration. The dexamethasone suppression test is increasingly employed by psychiatrists and other physicians to document depression in their patients. However, there are many false positive and negative responses in this test and its use as a reliable diagnostic marker is doubtful. Normal circadian rhythms involving

---

[36]The major action of chlorpromazine and the other phenothiazines is to block some of the excess dopamine receptors within the thalamus of schizophrenic patients. This is associated with a reduction of psychotic symptoms and signs. Such agents are rarely used in treating non-psychotic disorders (other than intractible nausea and vomiting and geriatric depression), but severe and agitated depression is an exception.

cortisol release are also different in depressed patients relative to controls. Cortisol release normally ceases during the evening and early morning, but is maintained in depressed persons; these abnormal profiles are restored to normal with remission of the depression. Chronically high levels of hydrocortisol due to norepinephrine deficits could feed into the interactions between it and serotonin described above (pages 78–79), resulting in serotonin depression and further cortisol elevation.

ANTIDEPRESSANT DRUGS

The first really effective drugs in the pharmacological armory for treating depression[37] were the *monoamine oxidase inhibitors (MAOI's)*. It was discovered that when patients with both tuberculosis and psychiatric depression were treated with the antitubercular drug, *isoniazid*, their depressions frequently remitted and they developed an elevated affect. About the same time it was learned that this and related compounds were effective inhibitors of monoamine oxidase, one of the enzymes which catabolizes both the catecholamines (DA and NE) and the indoleamines (serotonin). Further tests revealed that isoniazid alleviates the symptoms of depression in non-tubercular patients, as well. The mood-elevating effect of the MAOI's is due to the increased availability of amine neurotransmitters, especially of norepinephrine and serotonin, at synapses and within presynaptic axon terminals in the CNS. This enhanced activity of NE and serotonin results from the inhibition of their metabolic breakdown by MAO within the synaptic cleft, allowing them to remain longer in the vicinity of their receptor sites and having the effect of increasing their activity. There is an approximate correlation between the potency of these agents in suppressing MAO activity and their antidepressant efficacy.

The MAOI's generate a feeling of well-being and elation as well as some elevation in motor activity, and some of these drugs have an amphetaminelike quality (Bowman & Rand 1980). Subsequent clinical experience suggests that MAOI's are more effective in alleviating reactive than endogenous depression, and they are largely restricted to use

---

[37]Antianxiety agents and sedative-hypnotics are only marginally and temporarily useful in assisting such patients over rough periods. They do not constitute an effective, long-term chemotherapy for depression or any other psychiatric disorder. However, they are widely and effectively used in the treatment of seizure disorders.

with such patients. Even here, however, they are not commonly employed because of a variety of sometimes dangerous side effects.[38]

In addition to suppressing MAO, the MAOI's are also very potent inhibitors of hepatic microsomal enzymes, and in fact they inhibit a very wide range of enzyme systems. The inhibitory effect the MAOI's exert upon liver microsomal activity causes a very powerful potentiation of the actions of those drugs and substances which are normally inactivated by the microsomal monooxygenases (see Light 1985). Such drugs include most of the barbiturates and other sedative-hypnotics, morphine, anti-histamines, phenothiazines and tricyclic antidepressants. Much more importantly, the MAOI's potentiate the activity of certain biogenic amines such as *tyramine* and *phenylethylamine* which are formed by the bacterial decarboxylation of the amino acids tyrosine and *phenyalanine*, respectively. These amines tend to replace norepinephrine in the synaptic vesicles within the axon terminals; the norepinephrine thus released from the synaptic vesicles exerts its usual action upon the postsynaptic receptor sites. These biogenic amines thus indirectly act as sympathomimetic amines, causing false transmission. Tyramine is highly concentrated in certain foods such as some, but not all, cheeses, certain wines (especially chianti), beers, chicken livers, chocolate, and certain preserved meat and fish products (pickled herring). Such foods, if eaten while MAOI's are also being taken, may precipitate a severe hypertensive crisis.

These biogenic amines are degraded by MAO (as are the very closely related catecholamines, dopamine and norepinephrine), and the inhibition of MAO by the MAOI's partly accounts for the potentiation of these substances. However, the vast proportion of such potentiation results from the suppression of the microsomal enzymes by the MAOI's. Some of these amine-MAOI and drug-MAOI interactions can be fatal. Of particular concern is the fatal hepatotoxic reaction which occurs in about one of every 5,000 to 10,000 patients treated with these agents (Bowman & Rand 1980). Although the hepatic toxic reaction has a relatively low incidence, the fatal outcome of those affected is high (about 20%). This response is an idiosyncratic one which results from the formation of

---

[38]Toxic interactions between MAOI's and other drugs and biogenic amine containing foods certainly do occur, occasionally with fatal results. However, some authors (Bowman & Rand 1980) believe these risks have been vastly overestimated and feel that they are still very useful therapeutic agents in treating depression.

highly reactive metabolic intermediates which bind covalently to macro-molecules in the hepatocytes, causing their destruction. It is for such reasons that the MAOI's are not commonly employed in current clinical practice (see footnote 38).

The first of the tricyclic antidepressants (TCA's) to appear was *imipramine* or *Tofranil.*® The TCA's are closely related to the phenothiazines, which have a similar three-ring structure, and like the latter, were developed from chemically related antihistamines. Because of the obvious relationship between the phenothiazines and imipramine, the latter was tested with mental patients. Although it had no effect with schizophrenic patients it was very beneficial with depressed patients. Figure 22 shows the structures and relationships between the phenothiazines and TCA's. The planes of the two phenyl rings in the phenothiazines intersect each other at a slight angle; in the case of the TCA's the angle is much greater. As a general rule for these two classes of drugs, the more nearly planar the rings are, the greater is the *neuroleptic* activity (neuroleptic refers to the antipsychotic activity of the phenothiazines). Conversely, the greater is the angle between the two phenyl rings, the greater is the antidepressant effect.

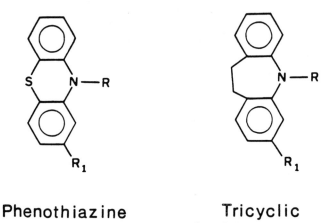

Phenothiazine   **Tricyclic Antidepressant**

Figure 22
Structures of Phenothiazines and Tricylcic Antidepressants

Like the phenothiazines, the TCA's both block the presynaptic reuptake of the catecholamines and indoleamines and they blockade the postsynaptic receptor sites for those neurotransmitters (Bowman & Rand 1980).

In the case of the phenothiazines, the postsynaptic blockade of the domanine receptors more than compensates for the suppression of dopamine reuptake by the presynaptic axon terminal, and the major effect is to depress the activity of that neurotransmitter. Because schizophrenia is associated with an excess number of dopamine receptors in the thalamus and corpus striatum, the inhibitory effect of the phenothiazines upon the receptors reduces the activity of dopamine, thus alleviating many of the psychotic symptoms. In the case of the TCA's, however, the blockage of neurotransmitter reuptake by the presynaptic terminals more than compensates for the blockade of the transmitter receptors. The major effect of the TCA's is thus to permit norepinephrine and, depending upon the specific drug, also serotonin to remain in the synaptic cleft for a longer than normal period. This overcomes the relative deficiencies of those transmitters and enhances their activity at the respective receptor sites. By thus compensating for the deficit of norepinephrine and serotonin, the symptoms of depression are relieved. The TCA's are also known to inhibit cyclic nucleotide phosphodiesterase (see above, figure 8). Because serotonin and norepinephrine operate by way of a two-messenger system (see figure 8) involving the generation of cAMP, deficits of either or both of those transmitters results in inadequate production of cAMP at the postsynaptic receptor sites. Inhibition of phosphodiesterase by TCA's allows that cAMP which is generated to remain longer in the postsynaptic system, thus enhancing its effects upon the membrane ionic gates. The closely related "tetracyclic" antidepressants (e.g. *maprotiline* or *Ludiomil*®) are thought to act in similar ways.

The profile of chemical activity of the TCA's can be altered by changing the structure slightly. *Secondary amines* are those TCA's that have only one methyl group ($-CH_3$) on the terminal nitrogen (see insert). Examples are *desipramine, nortriptyline* and *protriptyline*. TCA's bearing two methyl groups on the terminal nitrogen are called *tertiary amines*. Examples of tertiary amines include *imipramine, amitriptyline* (e.g. *Elavil*®), *doxepin, clomipramine* and *trimipramine*. The monomethylated or secondary amines block the uptake of norepinephrine and serotonin equally; the dimethylated or tertiary amines selectively block serotonin uptake relative to norepinephrine. In general, patients whose depression is caused primarily by norepinephrine deficiency (for the most part, so-called endogenous depressives) respond well to the monomethylated TCA's. Those depressed patients also presenting anger, agitation and early (as opposed to terminal) insomnia[39] are thought by some clinicians to be largely due to serotonin deficiency. These patients are generally much more responsive to the dimethylated amines.

The tricyclic antidepressants also appear to alter the rate of dopamine synthesis. Carlsson & Lindqvist (1978) reported that the secondary amines appear to decrease the rate of dopamine synthesis, perhaps because of the adjustment of the feedback response of the presynaptic autoreceptors in the face of prolonged neurotransmitter activity in the synaptic cleft. Tertiary amines, on the other hand, appear to enhance the rate of dopamine synthesis. Given the broad and complex symptomatology of depressive disorders it seems likely that the biochemical factors involved are far more intricate than we now suspect. Nevertheless, the fact that we can pharmacologically intervene in the affective disorders so effectively is in itself compelling evidence that the basic biochemical model generally agreed upon is accurate insofar as it goes.

The precise manner in which these drugs work remains largely obscure, however. Among the most puzzling aspects of TCA pharmacodynamics is the length of time after the initiation of TCA therapy for any clinical effects to become manifest. A lag period of three or four weeks is quite usual, and many patients discontinue the drug before it becomes effective because of the mild, but temporary side effects that commonly occur—especially anticholinergic effects such as "dry mouth," and more rarely, constipation, blurred vision, urinary retention and, occasionally,

---

[39]Inability to fall asleep after one has gone to bed at an appropriate time is called *early insomnia;* it is characteristic of reactive depression and "atypical" depression. Awakening very early in the morning long before one wishes to arise and being unable to get back to sleep is termed *terminal insomnia.* It is the characteristic insomnia of endogenous depression.

impotence. This lag period occurs despite adequate blood levels of the antidepressant. Two possibilities have been suggested (Bowman & Rand 1980): (1) the drug concentration at the specific target regions in the brain are accumulated only slowly; (2) the drug effect in the target regions is perhaps due to an alteration of neurotransmitter processes, and this effect is produced slowly. As in the case of the phenothiazines, individual responses to a given TCA are very idiosyncratic and it is often necessary to try two or three different types with an individual patient before one is found that is really effective. Furthermore, the various individual responses to these drugs are not predictable on the basis of a given set of symptoms or presumed diagnosis. The long lag period exhibited by many of these agents, and the fact that the dose must usually be built up over several weeks and likewise withdrawn only gradually, causes some patients to give up in despair. But with perseverance on the part of the patient and the physician, an adequate antidepressant can generally be found. The newer tetracyclic antidepressants appear to be effective in a much shorter time, often within a week or less, and they do not have as many side effects as the tricyclics. Furthermore, they are generally more effective in cases of so-called neurotic or reactive depression than are the tricyclics; in some cases they are approved by the FDA for such use.

Very recently a new class antidepressants derived from *triazolopyridine* have become available (e.g. *trazodone* or *Desyrel*®). These are chemically quite unrelated to the tricyclic, tetracyclic or other known antidepressants and they appear to have a faster onset of action and produce fewer side effects.

Finally, a comment about *electroconvulsive therapy (ECT)* or "shock treatment" for the treatment of intractable depression is in order, especially since there is much ignorance and prejudice about this approach. In current practice the patient is always lightly anaesthetized and given a short-acting muscle relaxant before ECT is given. This eliminates the unpleasant aspects of the treatment, and because there is no violent muscle contraction in response to the shock, bone fracture is now extremely rare. Death is an infrequent occurrence with from 3 to 9 deaths per 100,000 treatments (Klein *et al.* 1980). Transient memory loss is common, typically lasting from 30 to 90 minutes after the shock is administered. Very rarely memory loss is persistent. A typical treatment course consists of a current of 200–1500 milliamps applied for 0.1–0.6 seconds (Bowman

& Rand 1980). This is repeated every few days until the symptoms are gone or until no further improvement is gained. By and large this treatment is very effective in relieving severe depression, often permanently. It is usually employed in cases where the patient has not responded to either TCA's or MAOI's and the depression is severe enough to warrant such treatment. The collective experience is that patients who do not respond to TCA's or MAOI's usually respond very well to ECT, and *vice versa*. ECT has been demonstrated to produce elevated levels of monoamines—especially of serotonin—in the brains of laboratory animals, and it is generally thought that this is the major mechanism by which it alleviates depression.

Mania, the opposite affective pole from depression, has already been briefly described, and it will be dealt with further in a later volume which discusses the genetic relationships between affective disorder and alcoholism. Mania is generally agreed upon as resulting at least in large measure from an excess of norepinephrine production at the adrenergic nerve terminals. Mania and hypomania are often very effectively treated with lithium salts, generally lithium carbonate or lithium chloride. Lithium is the lightest of the metals and it is closely related to sodium and potassium. Although it was discovered in Australia in 1949 to be effective in the treatment of manic disorders, it was not widely prescribed for that purpose in this country prior to 1970. Lithium rarely occurs endogenously in biological systems and it has no known nontherapeutic physiological functions. When administered its volume of distribution (see Light 1985) corresponds roughly to that of the total body water, that is, it does not strongly segregate into the various body-water compartments (plasma water, extracellular and intracellular fractions). However, there are higher concentrations of lithium in the intracellular water of the brain relative to the interstitial (extracellular) water, these being on the order of 4:2. The situation is reversed in other organ systems (Klein *et al.* 1980). Within the brain, lithium becomes relatively more concentrated at the nerve terminals than elsewhere. Increases in the extracellular concentration of both sodium and lithium ions increases the rate of neuronal uptake of norepinephrine. When used in the treatment of mania, lithium ions facilitate the uptake of norepinephrine by central (and peripheral) adrenergic neurons, thus decreasing its availability and countering its manic effects. It appears to be equally effective in treating both "unipolar" manic[40] patients and bipolar depressed patients. In view of the current model describing mania as resulting from a norepinephrine excess and depression from a norepinephrine and/or serotonin deficit, the mechanism by which lithium suppresses both mania and depression in bipolar patients remains obscure. Lithium, like the TCA's, has a delayed onset of efficacy—generally one to two weeks. Gastrointestinal and neurological side effects are not uncommon, the former including pain, loss of appetite, thirst, nausea and vomiting, and diarrhea. Among the neurological effects are dizziness, tremor, ataxia (loss of motor coordination), muscular twitching and slurred speech. Dangerous toxic effects appear with doses very close to the required therapeutic dose and careful monitoring of the patient is required.

ALCOHOL AND THE BRAIN

Drugs can affect nervous transmission in the brain in a number of ways:

(1) by packing into the phospholipid bilayer, thus fluidizing and distorting the architecture of neural membranes and altering membrane permeability.

(2) by affecting the binding of Ca^{++} to the gangliosides along neural membranes, thus impairing the operation of the Na^+ and K^+ ionic gates.

(3) by interfering with the action potential as it invades the presynaptic terminal.

(4) by inhibiting the influx of Ca^{++} into the presynaptic terminal, thus impairing the fusion of the synaptic vesicles to the presynaptic membrane and interfering with the release of neurotransmitter into the synaptic cleft.

(5) by interfering with the uptake of precursor molecules at the axon terminal needed to synthesize neurotransmitters (such as choline and the amino acids tyrosine and tryptophan).

(6) by interfering with the synthesis of the transmitter.

(7) by interfering with the storage of neurotransmitter in the presynaptic vesicles (as occurs with certain condensation products of monoamines and aldehydes generated by ethanol oxidation).

(8) by altering postsynaptic membrane permeability.

---

[40] By definition, mania is a *bipolar* illness. As used here, "unipolar" refers to those cases of bipolar disorder presenting only manic episodes.

(9) by blocking or activating postsynaptic receptor sites—i.e., by acting as an antagonist or an agonist.

(10) by interfering with presynaptic receptors.

(11) by interfering with the second messenger system.

(12) by affecting the rate at which neurotransmitters are removed from the synaptic cleft: (a) by action on degradative enzymes, and (b) by action on the presynaptic reuptake mechanisms.

Ethanol causes increased binding of calcium and magnesium ions, which competetively inhibits Na^+ influx during nerve firing. It has been demonstrated by several investigators (Noble & Tewari 1978) that ethanol does in fact inhibit Na^+ influx during nerve firing. It also restricts the reuptake of K^+ during the recovery or refractory phase. The inhibition of Na^+ influx because of increased membrane fluidity, causing ionic stereochemical distortion or inhibition of the sodium gates, and increased calcium binding appear to be critical factors in the depression of the CNS due to alcohol, and the direct inhibition of nervous impulses is almost certainly a major consequence. Calcium ions are also involved in the release of neurotransmitters from the axon terminals. Increased binding of Ca^{++} in these regions would also interfere with synaptic transmission.

Ethanol is also known to inhibit the phosphate-cleaving enzyme, *adenosinetriphosphatase* or *ATPase* (see above, pages 8–10 and figure 5). Such inhibition would restrict the operation of the ATP-dependent sodium-potassium pump, thereby diminishing the rate at which outward-leaking potassium ions are returned to the intracellular medium and reducing the resting potential of the neural membrane. This effect appears to be a secondary result of the general membrane disruption that occurs with ethanol administration, rather than a primary factor in the CNS changes induced by the drug. Indeed, the major effect of reduced $[Na^+ - K^+]$-activated ATPase levels and the consequent lowered resting potential would appear to be one of *facilitation*[41] rather than inhibition of nervous transmission. There is evidence that alcohol in small amounts can have a direct excitatory effect on neuronal activity, whereas larger amounts of the drug suppress such effects. This initial excitement is probably due to the inhibition of the sodium-potassium pump and the consequent lowering of the resting membrane potential which increases membrane permeability. By increasing membrane fluidity (see below) alcohol also increases the

---

[41]In facilitation, the threshold intensity of the stimulus required to initiate an action potential or the degree of stimulation needed to elicit a given level of a graded potential is reduced, and the generation of such an impulse is thus enhanced.

tendency for synaptic vesicles to fuse with the presynaptic membrane. This results in enhanced spontaneous release of the transmitter into the synaptic cleft. It thus appears that not all of the "excitement" in the early stages of intoxication is "paradoxical" (see also above, pages 82–83). At least some of it may also reflect a genuine neurological stimulation. This early facilitation of nervous transmission due to low ethanol doses is soon overwhelmed by the much stronger inhibitory effects of membrane fluidization seen at larger doses.

All animal cells are surrounded by a *plasma membrane*. The membranes surrounding a neuron is called a *neural membrane* or *neurolemma*. Such membranes are composed of a double layer of *phospholipids* (molecules in which two fatty acids are linked to a glycerol frame, with the third methylene group of the glycerol being occupied by a highly polar phosphate group; see Light 1985 for a more detailed explanation). The polar phosphate heads are attracted to the polar water molecules in the cellular and extracellular media, whereas the nonpolar fatty-acid tails are repelled by the water. This results in their spontaneous arrangement into two layers with the polar heads directed outwards towards the watery environment and the nonpolar tails pointing inward (figure 3). Scattered within this phospholipid bilayer are various proteins which function as enzymes, structural units, or which serve as carrier molecules in transporting other lipid insoluble molecules across the membrane. This is illustrated in figure 23A.

The membrane proteins also tend to be amphipathic and are partially embedded in and partially protruding from the lipid bilayer. Those protruding portions of the integral proteins contain the ionic residues of the respective amino acids, whereas the embedded protein fractions are mainly nonpolar. Cholesterol molecules are also embedded in the membrane system in various places. The many different types of membrane proteins selectively bind to specific membrane lipids, and the former, being genetically coded, may specify the types and ratios of the membrane lipids (Bowman & Rand 1980). The fatty acid tails of the phospholipids contain both saturated and unsaturated residues. The degree of membrane fluidity, that is, the orderly packing of the fatty acid tails and the relative freedom of the membrane proteins to move laterally within the bilayer, is determined by the number of unsaturated ($-C = C-$) bonds and length of the fatty acid tails, and the amount of cholesterol present in the system. The unsaturated carbon bonds alter the shape of the hydrocarbon chains and result in a less orderly packing arrangement of the fatty acid tails (figure 23A). The greater the number of unsaturated bonds, the greater is the disorder (fluidity) of the membrane architecture, and the greater is the freedom of movement of the embedded proteins. Cholesterol, however, forms stable complexes with unsaturated fatty acids, restoring normal membrane architecture and causing the membrane to become more rigid and crystallized.

Ethanol has weak polar ($-OH$) and nonpolar groups; it is therefore simultaneously both hydrophilic and hydrophobic, that is it is *amphipathic.* It readily passes through aqueous channels or pores in cell membranes, and is in fact distributed throughout the body water (see the section on the volume of distribution in Light 1985). But because it is also lipid soluble (the partition ratio between tissue lipids and tissue water is about 25:1; see footnote 43) it is not confined solely to the aqueous phase at the water-lipid interfaces of neural membranes. Ethanol also packs into the lipid portion of neural membranes and disrupts their orderly arrangement (figure 23B). The distortion in membrane architecture sterochemically interferes with the normal operation of ionic gate proteins, inhibiting ionic flux and interfering with neural transmission. While the nonpolar, lipophlic part of the ethanol molecule fluidizes the superficial lipid portion of the membrane, the polar moiety may also interact with the ionic charges of the protruding portions of the membrane proteins (figure 23B). This could result in an alteration of the charge distributions of those proteins, thus causing further conformational changes and/or otherwise inhibiting their normal functioning still further.

The increase in membrane fluidity separates the lipid molecules from one another and permits greater lateral movement of membrane components. Fluid membranes are more likely to spontaneously fuse with one another, and this may result in increased fusion of neurotransmitter-containing vesicles with the presynaptic membrane in axon terminals (Littleton 1980). The resulting increase in transmitter release into the synaptic cleft may contribute to the initial neuronal excitement produced by low to moderate doses of ethanol (see above, page 82). Because brain synaptic membranes have a high number of polyunsaturated phospholipid fatty acid tails, the action of alcohol may be particularly pronounced at the synapse. Higher doses of alcohol may affect the binding of agonist molecules to their receptors in the membrane, and the increased lateral mobility of membrane proteins due to membrane expansion may cause the decoupling of receptors and their associated enzymes such as adenylate cyclase (see figure 24). This would tend to depress normal neural functioning.

However, the composition of membrane lipids, and thus also membrane fluidity, is carefully controlled by adjusting the proportions of

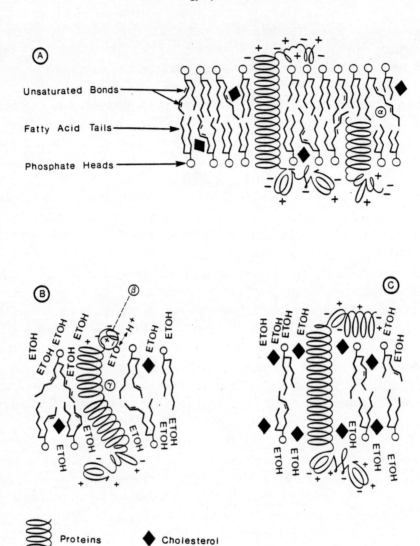

Unsaturated Bonds

Fatty Acid Tails

Phosphate Heads

Proteins   ◆ Cholesterol

Figure 23

The Action of Ethanol on Membrane Architecture

Cell membranes consist of a phospholipid bilayer. The covalent and hydrophobic fatty acid tails are directed away from both the extracellular and intracellular water, whereas the polar phosphate heads are attracted inwardly and outwardly toward the water fractions. A variety of integral proteins are embedded within and partially protruding from the membrane bilayer. The protruding portions of the proteins contain the charged, ionic residues (+ and −). In contrast, the nonpolar residues are largely embedded within the lipid bilayer where they tend to assume typical alpa helical configurations. Membrane fluidity is determined by the number of unsaturated carbon bonds on the phospholipid fatty acid tails, as well as by the amount of cholesterol present. Unsaturated fatty acids create a structural deformation resulting in a less orderly packing arrangement of the phospholipid molecules. Cholesterol forms stable complexes with unsaturated fatty acids, thus immobilizing the membranes and making them more rigid.

A. Normal membrane structure and fluidity permitting some mobility of the component proteins which variously serve as ionic gates, enzymes, carrier proteins and structural units. A moderate number of unsaturated fatty acids resulting in moderate membrane expansion (a); this fluidity is slightly countered by occasional cholesterol molecules which form stable hydrophobic complexes with the carbon double bonds. This results in an optimal state of membrane fluidity commensurate with normal functioning. B. The covalent portions of ethanol molecules are packed into the superficial portions of the lipid bilayer causing membrane expansion and increasing the distances between membrane components (γ). The resulting structural distortion interferes with the proper functioning of integral proteins. Protein configuration and thus their function is further compromised by the tendency of the polar hydroxyl groups of the alcohol molecules to interact with charged protein residues protruding from the lipid bilayer (β). C. Membrane adaptation to the fluidizing effects of ethanol are brought about by a significant reduction in the amount of unsaturation in the fatty acid tails, as well as by significant increases in the amount of membrane cholesterol. This makes the membranes more rigid and tends to restore normal neural functioning. Elevated cholesterol levels tend to exclude alcohol molecules from the bilayer.

Short-chain alcohols like ethanol are restricted to the surface layers of membrane systems since their covalent, lipid-soluble portions are very small and the polar effects of the hydroxyl groups relatively strong. More massive alcohols correspondingly penetrate deeper into the lipid bilayer causing structural deformation at more profound levels.

---

saturated and unsaturated fatty acids in the lipid bilayer by the cells. This bilayer responds to a sustained ethanol challenge by reducing the number of double bonds near the surface of the membrane (Littleton 1980). This results in decreased membrane fluidity and increased orderliness of the packing arrangement in the lipid bilayer. Membrane cholesterol content is also greatly increased (figure 23C), further stabilizing the membrane and decreasing the extent of alcohol binding. Indeed, the increase in cholesterol content appears to be quantitatively more important in enhancing membrane stability than the reduction in unsaturated fatty acid bonds.

The ethanol-induced fluidizing effect and accompanying architectural distortion of neural membranes appear to be the major mechanisms involved in the development of pharmacological tolerance. Chronic ethanol administration in rats causes increased resistance by brain membranes to the structural alterations known to be produced by the drug.[42] Under prolonged ethanol insult, the neural membranes develop a greater rigidity and corresponding resistance to the increased fluidity induced by alcohol in controls.[43] Furthermore, this resistance to ethanol-dis-

---

[42](Rottenberg et al. 1981). This same resistance is also found in the membranes of the liver cell mitochondria.

[43]As the membrane becomes more fluid, the *partitioning coefficient* of ethanol becomes correspondingly greater, resulting in its enhanced uptake and binding by the membrane system. The partitioning coefficient, B = concentration of substance in oil ÷ its concentration in water, is a measure of a compound's relative solubilities in lipids and water. The higher the partitioning coefficient, the greater is its solubility in lipid and vice versa.

ordering also extends to the structural disordering produced by halothane (an inhalant general anaesthetic) as well as to that due to phenobarbitol. In fact, the neural membranes from ethanol-adapted rats are much more rigid than are normal membranes which have not been exposed to ethanol, and they become as fluid as those of normal animals *only in the presence of moderate concentrations of ethanol!* The normal state of fluidity is considered to be optimal for proper function of the system. The authors of the paper reporting this phenomenon (Rottenburg *et al.* 1981) suggest that the excessive rigidity of the neural membranes of ethanol-adapted rats underlies the twin phenomena of tolerance and physical dependency, since these tissues appear only to function optimally in the presence of significant amounts of alcohol. In the authors' own words:[44] " . . . chronic consumption of ethanol induces an . . . increased membrane rigidity (decreased fluidity), which leads to a reduction in the binding of alcohol- . . . and to the acquisition of tolerance. The increased rigidity impairs normal membrane function in the absence of ethanol, but [with] . . . moderate concentrations of ethanol the membrane becomes sufficiently fluid to resemble normal membranes (dependence). Since the membrane is more rigid it also binds fewer molecules of anesthetics (cross-tolerance)."

The mechanism by which membrane adaptation to chronic ethanol challenge becomes "fixed" so that it cannot return to its previous normal state of fluidity, thus producing physical dependency upon the drug, is not known at this time. However, two possibilities have been suggested by Littleton (1980):

(1) Fatty acid turnover and thus alteration in the ratio of saturated to. unsaturated bonds may become significantly slowed as dependency increases; this would impair the ability of rapid response to ethanol withdrawal and perpetuate a hyperrigid state characterized by a more or less stable reduction in the number of unsaturated fatty acid bonds.

(2) With continued ethanol challenge, short-term adaptive responses such as changes in fatty acid composition may be replaced by other changes which cannot be readily reversed, such as alterations in membrane proteins or phospholipid head groups.

Fatty acid transport into the mitochondria in all cells for beta-oxidation is dependent upon carnitine (see figure 21 in Light 1985). Carnitine may also be involved for the transport of fatty acids across neuronal membranes. It has been demonstrated that ethanol-treated rats require higher than

---

[44]Rottenburg *et al.* 1981: 584.

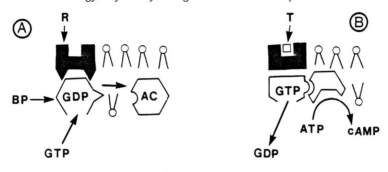

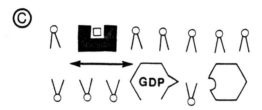

Figure 24
Membrane Fluidization and the Adenylate Cyclase System

The second-messenger adenylate cyclase system by which postsynaptic potentials are generated is actually more complex than indicated in figure 8 and the corresponding portions of the text. In fact the adenylate cyclase system is activated by an intermediate protein which binds guanosine triphosphate (GTP). The resting state of the receptor-adenylate cyclase system is shown in A. In B the activating neurotransmitter (T) binds to the receptor, R, causing it to undergo a configurational change; guanosine diphosphate (GDP) is released from the binding protein (BP) and replaced by GTP. BP is activated by GTP and moves laterally within the membrane lipid system and binds to the adenylate cyclase complex (AC). The latter is activated and converts ATP into cAMP, which then activates a kinase, which in turn phosphorylates a membrane ionic gate (see also figure 8). Normal membrane function requires a certain amount of lateral mobility of proteins within the lipid bilayer. With excessive membrane fluidization such as occurs with an ethanol challenge (C) the lateral mobility of membrane proteins may become so pronounced that receptor-binding protein-enzyme complexes are dissociated, thus interfering with the functioning of these systems. Modified and expanded from Schramm & Selinger 1984).

normal levels of carnitine to effect mitochondrial beta-oxidation of fatty acids. Furthermore, carnitine translocase, the enzyme which carries carnitine:fatty acid complexes across membranes, appears to be inhibited by chronic administration of ethanol (Reitz 1977 *in* Littleton 1980). Abu Murad and his colleagues (1977) have also demonstrated that increased dietary intake of carnitine dramatically alleviates ethanol-induced physical withdrawal in mice. Carnitine may therefore play a significant role in the development of membrane physical dependence to alcohol.

Tetrahydroisoquinolines and Alcohol

The oxidation of large amounts of ethanol *in vivo* can also interfere with the normal degradation of the catecholamines and serotonin. Both dopamine and norepinephrine are converted into their respective aldehyde derivatives, both by monoamine oxidase acting alone, and by the combined action of MAO and catechol-O-methyltransferase (figures 9B and 25). Serotonin is similarly broken down into 5-hydroxindole-3-acetaldehyde by MAO alone and acting in concert with 5-hydroxyindole-O-methyltransferase (5-HIOMT) (see figure 9C). These aminealdehydes are then either reduced into their respective alcohols by alcohol dehydrogenase accompanied by the oxidation of NADH plus H^+ into NAD^+, or they are oxidized into their one or more derivative acids by aldehyde dehydrogenase, along with the reduction of NAD^+ into NADH plus H^+ (see figures 9B–C, 25, and 26). Dopamine, for example, is ultimately metabolized into either its alcohol, 3-methoxy-4-hydroxyphenylethanol (MOPET), or into homovanillic acid (HVA) (figure 25).

The metabolic pathway for alcohol oxidation, most of which occurs in the liver, is:

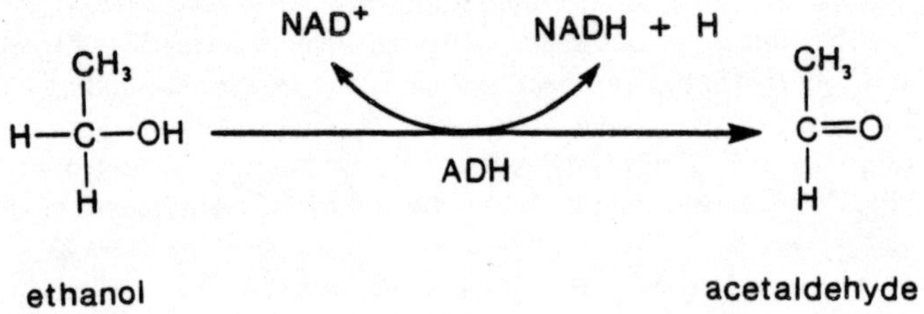

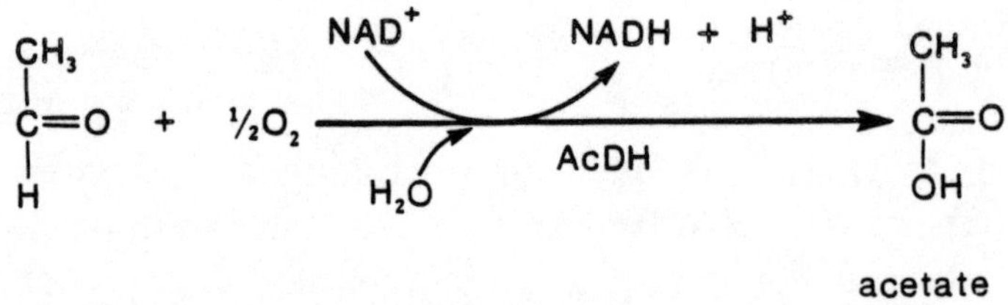

The mass effect of large amounts of acetaldehyde resulting from ethanol oxidation outcompetes the aminealdehyde for the enzyme aldehyde dehydrogenase, thereby blocking the conversion of the aminealdehyde into its acid derivative (figure 26). The pathway is therefore shifted to favor the conversion of the aminealdehyde into its alcohol. The excess of reducing equivalents generated by ethanol and acetaldehyde oxidation (see Light 1985 for a detailed discussion of this) also inhibit the oxidation of the aminealdehyde into its acid, and favor its reduction into the alcohol. However, the high concentration of ethanol outcompetes the aminealdehyde for the enzyme alcohol dehydrogenase. There is a net buildup, therefore, of both aminealdehydes and acetaldehyde. Both of these aldehydes can then form condensation products with endogenous catecholamines and indolealkyamines (figure 27).

Condensation reactions are broadly defined as a series of non-enzymatic, spontaneous reactions involving amine ($-NH_2$) and carbonyl ($-C=O$) compounds (*i.e.*, aldehydes or a-keto acids) in equilibrium with the first condensation product—an *aldimine compound* or *Schiff's* base. Thus:

$$
\begin{array}{cc}
R & R \\
| & | \\
NH_2 \quad \xrightarrow{\text{amine compound}} & N \\
\rightleftharpoons & \| \\
 & HC \\
HC=O \quad \text{carbonyl compound} & | \\
| & \\
R & R
\end{array}
\quad \text{Schiff's base}
$$

Under certain circumstances these condensation products can form irreversible, secondarily cyclic (heterocyclic)[45] compounds (see figure 27A–D). If the starting amino-compound is a phenylethylamine (see above, page 22) such as dopamine, the condensation products formed will be *tetrahydroisoquinolines* (THIQ's). If the starting amino-compounds are indolethylamines (indolealkylamines, see above, page 23) such as tryptophan or its tryptamine derivatives (including serotonin), the condensation products will be *tetrahydro-beta-carbolines* (Collins 1980). The THIQ's are in the biosynthetic pathway leading to the *anhalonia alkaloids* such as *mescaline, hordenine, pellotine, anhalonidine, lophophorine, anhalonine, anhalamine* and *anhalinine* from the peyotl or peyote cactus, *Lophophora williamsii* [=*Anhalonium lewinii*]. The powerful psychedelic properties of these substances are well known. The tetrahydro-beta-carbolines are in the biosynthetic pathway to the *harmala alkaloids* which contain the serotonin skeleton within their structures and which are chemically

---

[45]The monoamine precursors as well as the aminealdehydes formed from them are already cyclic compounds. Their condensation products tend to form secondarily more complex cyclic, or heterocyclic compounds.

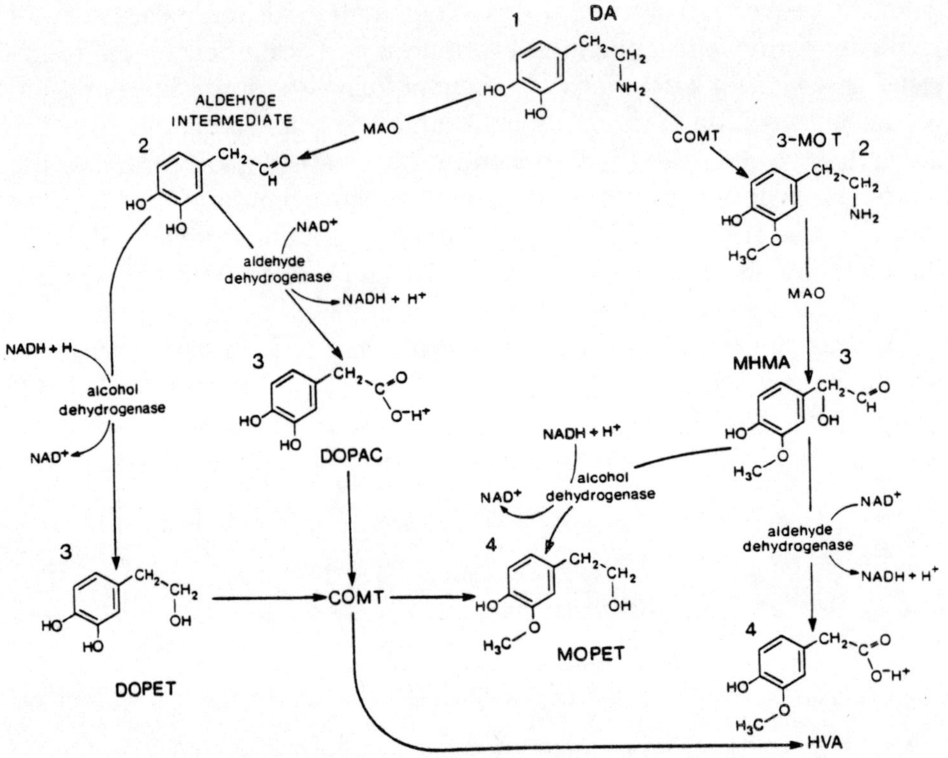

Figure 25
Combined Action of MAO and COMT on Dopamine

Monoamine oxidase (MAO) and catechol-O-methyltransferase (COMT) act in concert in very much the same way upon catecholamines (dopamine and norepinephrine). Serotonin undergoes very similar transformations by MAO and 5-hydroxyindole-O-methyltransferase. Dopamine (1) is converted by MAO into its aldehyde intermediate (2 on lefthand side of figure). The aldehyde is then either reduced into its alcohol, 3, 4-dihydroxyphenylethanol (DOPET), or oxidized into its acid, 3, 4-dihydroxyphenylacetic acid (DOPAC). Dopamine is converted by COMT into 3-methoxytyramine (3-MOT) (2 on the righthand side of the figure), which is subsequently changed into its aldehyde, 3-methoxy-4-hydroxymethylaldehyde (MHMA). MHMA is then reduced into the alcohol 3-methoxy-4-hydroxyphenylethanol (MOPET) or oxidized into homovanillic acid (HVA) [=3-methoxy-4-hydroxyphenylacetic acid]. DOPET is further metabolized via COMT into MOPET, and DOPAC is converted by COMT to HVA. (See also above, figure 9.) Modified from Bowman & Rand 1980.

closely related to LSD-25 and to psilocybin and related psychoactive agents.[46]

---

[46]Both the lysergide-type (indolealkylamines) and the mescaline-type (phenylethylamines) condensation products act as MAO inhibitors. In addition, the lysergide-type condensates blockade the serotonin receptors in the raphe nuclei and thus indirectly stimulate the reticular activating system by inhibitory release.

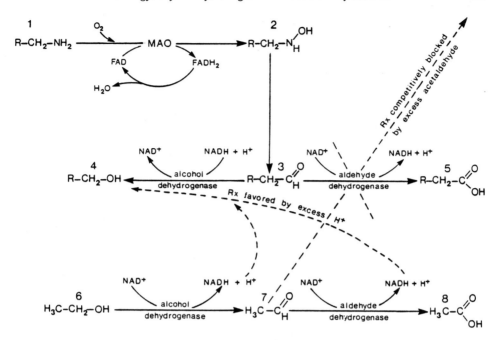

Figure 26
Inhibition of Monoamine Metabolism by Ethanol

Monoamine oxidase catalyzes the oxidative deamination of catecholamines and other amines in a process in which FAD is reduced to $FADH_2$ and oxygen is absorbed and a water molecule given off. The amine precursor (1) is first converted into its intermediate hydroxylamine (2). The intermediate is then converted into an aldehyde (3), a transient metabolite which then undergoes one of two reactions: (a) oxidation by aldehyde dehydrogenase into its acid (5) or (b) reduction into its alcohol (4). When large amounts of ethanol (6) are metabolized, the mass effect of the resulting acetaldehyde (7) outcompetes the aminealdehyde for the enzyme aldehyde dehydrogenase, and blocks the conversion of that amine metabolite into its acid form; (8) = acetate. The generation of excess reducing equivalents consequent to ethanol and acetaldehyde oxidation compounds the inhibition of the oxidation of the amine-aldehyde, and also favors its reduction into the alcohol form. But because of the competition between ethanol and the amine-aldehyde for alcohol dehydrogenase, there is a net buildup of both the aminealdehyde and acetaldehyde. Both aldehydes can then form condensation products with naturally occurring catecholamine and indoleamine neurotransmitters. Modified from Bowman & Rand, 1980.

Dopamine and acetaldehyde generated from the oxidation of ethanol condense to form *salsolinol* (figure 27A), a substance thought to act as a false transmitter substance in central catecholaminergic neurons. More importantly, dopamine and its own aldehyde metabolite condense to form *tetrahydropapaveroline* (figure 27B), a potent beta-adrenoreceptor agonist.[47] Tetrahydropapaveroline is also a precursor molecule in the

---

[47]This action can result in tremor, accelerated pulse and hypotension; this response may also mediate some of the hangover effects due to alcohol.

biosynthetic pathway for morphine and other opiate alkaloids in the opium poppy and a similar transformation may occur within dopamine-rich regions of the brain (Bowman & Rand 1980). An opiate-like physical dependence involving the endogenous opiate receptors may be one of the consequences of prolonged ethanol abuse.

THIQ's interact with the synaptic mechanisms involved in catecholamine activity in a number of ways (Cohen 1979). THIQ's and catecholamines compete for the transport sites on the presynaptic axonal membrane and in the presynaptic catecholamine storage vesicles. As a result the THIQ's competitively block the presynaptic reuptake of catecholamine neurotransmitters and are preferentially taken up and stored in the presynaptic catecholamine vesicles. Because of these actions, THIQ's are released from the nerve terminals along with the naturally occurring catecholamines by the series of events resulting from the entry of an action potential into the axon terminal. In addition, THIQ's induce the spontaneous release of endogenous catecholamines from the axon terminals into the synaptic cleft, probably by competitive displacement of the latter from the synaptic vesicles. They interact with the postsynaptic catecholamine receptor sites, and as previously mentioned, also function as MAO inhibitors and further inhibit presynaptic catecholamine reuptake. Although the THIQ's exert only a weak inhibition upon MAO relative to many other MAO inhibitors, their tendency to be stored in the presynaptic vesicles concentrates their intraneuronal antagonistic effects upon MAO, resulting in a strong inhibition upon that enzyme system. The increased residue of naturally occurring dopamine and norepinephrine within the nerve terminals permits an enhanced release of these neurotransmitters into the synaptic cleft due to their displacement by the THIQ's. The THIQ's are not themselves substrates for the action of MAO.

THIQ's are known to cause competetive feedback inhibition of tyrosine hydroxylase (see figure 9B) which catalyzes the conversion of tyrosine into L-dopa. This prevents the synthesis of both dopamine and norepinephrine within the nerve terminals, causing eventual depletion of both of those catecholamines. Catecholamine-derived THIQ's can act either agonistically or antagonistically upon a variety of receptors and tissues, depending upon the target sites and the particular THIQ involved. They thus act as *false* or *surrogate neurotransmitters* which can variously activate or blockade specific catecholamine receptors. They directly pro-

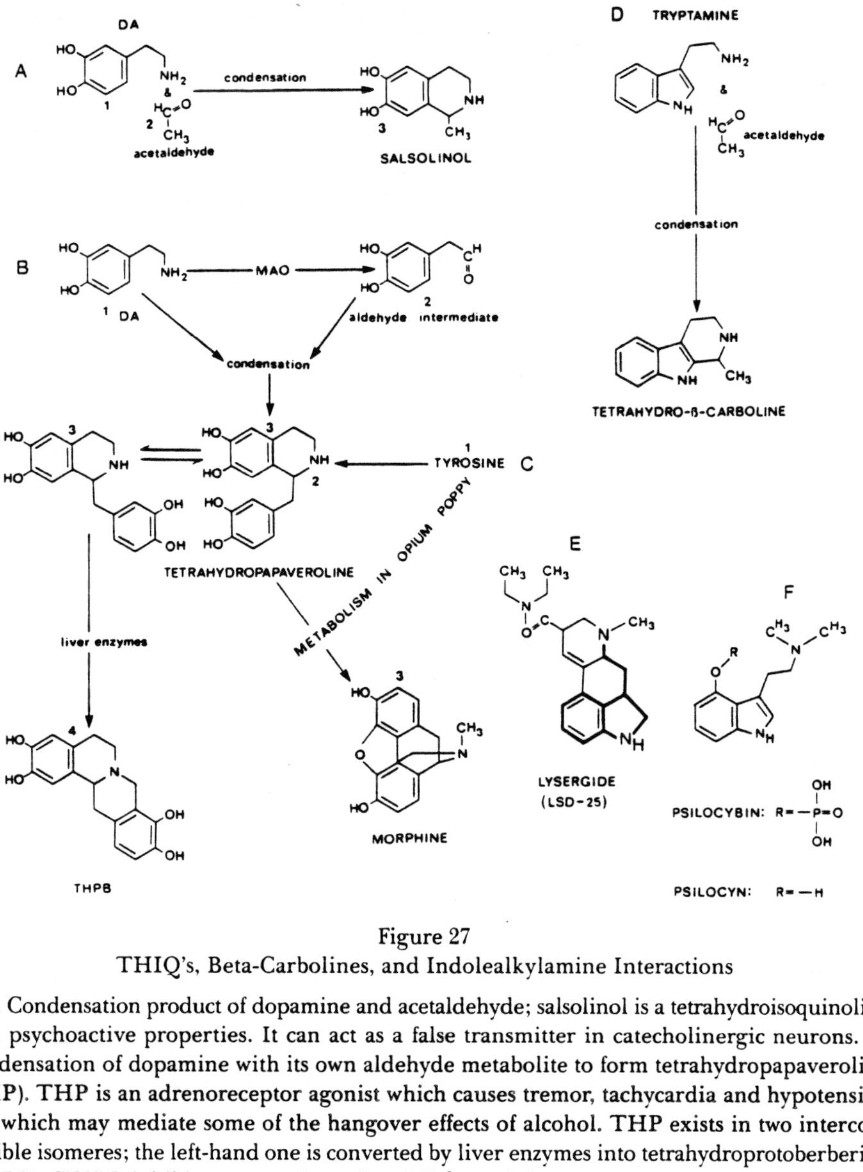

Figure 27
THIQ's, Beta-Carbolines, and Indolealkylamine Interactions

A. Condensation product of dopamine and acetaldehyde; salsolinol is a tetrahydroisoquinoline with psychoactive properties. It can act as a false transmitter in catecholinergic neurons. B. Condensation of dopamine with its own aldehyde metabolite to form tetrahydropapaveroline (THP). THP is an adrenoreceptor agonist which causes tremor, tachycardia and hypotension and which may mediate some of the hangover effects of alcohol. THP exists in two interconvertible isomeres; the left-hand one is converted by liver enzymes into tetrahydroprotoberberine (THBP). THBP inhibits neuronal uptake of Ca^{2+} and depresses the activity of ATPases; it also interacts directly with dopaminergic receptors. C. The pathway by which morphine is naturally synthesized in the opium poppy; THP is an intermediate step, and a similar conversion may occur in DA-rich regions of the brain. D. Condensation of tryptophan (and also of serotonin) with acetaldehyde to form psychoactive tetrahydro-β-carbolines. E. LSD-25: the heavy lines elucidate the serotonin skeleton. F. Psilocybin and Psilocyn: the indolealkylamine skeleton is obvious. Tetrahydro-β-carbolines, lysergide and the psilocybinlike compounds produce psychoactive effects by interacting with serotonin receptors in the CNS. The numbers indicate the sequence of reactions in pathways B and C.

mote lipolysis in the adipose reserves and can thus contribute to the hyperlipemia and fatty liver buildup consequent to ethanol intake (see Light 1985).

Salsolinol-type THIQ's significantly increase ethanol-induced sleep time in mice even when the ethanol is administered a full week after a single intraventricular injection[48] of the salsolinol. The sleep time is increased by nearly two and a half times (Melchior 1980). Condensation products formed from epinephrine and acetaldehyde cause a number of ultrastructural alterations and degenerative changes in the adrenergic nerve terminals within rat heart tissue (Oswald & Azevedo 1980). Among these changes are the following:

(1) increased axoplasmic density;
(2) decreased number or total absence of synaptic vesicles;
(3) disruption of the nerve microtubles involved in axoplasmic transport;
(4) altered and anomalous mitochondria;
(5) more severely damaged nerve terminals exhibit a thick packing of dense bodies and a degeneration of the entire terminals.

Neighboring Schwann cells within the rat auricles show indentations of the nuclear surface, multiplicity of ribosomes and very prominent rough endoplasmic reticulum and Golgi bodies. The Schwann cells tend to send off cytoplasmic processes which engulf and digest the damaged nerves. The neurotoxic properties of at least some THIQ's are thus clear.

Perhaps the most intriguing implications for the role played by ethanol-induced THIQ action in the brain come from behavioral studies with rats. When rats are given chronic intraventricular injections of dopamine-derived THIQ's, in particular salsolinol, their consumption of ethanol is vastly increased over that of controls (Cohen 1979; Melchior 1980). This increase in ethanol intake occurs despite the fact that high doses of ethanol are normally aversive to such rats and that the ethanol concentrations were increased from 3% to 30% over a 12-day period. The ethanol consumption rose to the point where the rats remained continually intoxicated—some rats drank as much as 13–16 grams of alcohol per day. The rats drank to the point of ataxia and some of

---

[48]Injection into the central or third ventricle of the brain.

them showed signs of physical withdrawal with tail stiffness, erection of the body hair and gross tremors. This effect of grossly increased ethanol consumption due to THIQ administration appears to be permanent, and the rats so treated continued to voluntarily consume very large amounts of alcohol for months after the treatment was discontinued (Melchior 1980).

Although the foregoing interactions between amine neurotransmitters and their condensation products with aldehydes has been well-documented by many *in vitro* studies, *in vivo* studies with laboratory animals have not unequivocally shown that THIQ's and beta-carbolines are generated in significant amounts by challenges with large amounts of ethanol alone (Noble & Teware 1978; Lieber 1982). Nevertheless, these condensation products do appear to be normal products in human metabolism and salsolinol and its O-methylated derivative and the methylated derivatives of 1-carbonyl-THP normally occur in human urine (Collins 1980). The last THIQ is also normally found in the human brain. Certain beta-carboline and aldehyde condensates also appear to build up naturally in human lens tissue as a function of the normal aging process. It has been shown (Collins 1980) that chronic drinking in alcoholics results in significant increases in urinary salsolinol and O-methyl-salsolinol, and that, indeed, these condensation products are generally increased during pathological states. The major mechanism underlying the increase in these metabolites in response to chronic, heavy alcohol intake appears to be due to the effects of acetaldehyde and aminealdehyde accumulation as described above.

Alcohol and Neurotransmitters

Despite the massive alterations in redox balances in the liver and other organs caused by the oxidation of large amounts of ethanol, no consistent redox shifts have been observed in the central nervous system due to the metabolism of alcohol (Christensen & Higgens 1979). Nevertheless, the excess of reducing equivalents which accumulate in the liver from alcohol metabolism depresses gluconeogenesis and, in conjunction with dietary inadequacies, can deprive the brain of the glucose necessary for its normal functioning. Ethanol also impairs the oxidation by the brain of that glucose which is still available. On the one hand this interferes still further with normal neuronal metabolism, and on the other this reduced utilization allows glucose to accumulate in these tissues (Reitz 1979). Both acute and chronic ethanol ingestion enhance the rate of glycogen breakdown by the brain which also contributes to the buildup of brain glucose following ethanol administration. The enhanced glycogenolysis appears to be due to catecholamine release resulting from the activation of the pituitary-adrenal axis by stressful doses of ethanol. The buildup of acetaldehyde following alcohol oxidation may also enhance brain glycogenolysis (Reitz 1979). The major factor behind decreased glucose utilization in the brain appears to be inhibition of the TCA cycle, probably primarily by the mass effect of acetyl co-A (see Light 1985) or perhaps because of disruption of the mitochondrial membrane architecture due to the general fluidizing effect of this drug. About 20% of the total oxygen consumption in a resting person occurs in the brain (White *et al.* 1978). When this rate of respiration is decreased because of reduced glucose supply to and/or utilization by the brain, cerebral function can be severely compromised.

Ethanol increases acetylcholine release in the motor end plates of neuromuscular junctions, possibly as a function of changes in membrane conductance and/or enhanced receptor sensitivity to the transmitter (Massarelli 1979). In contrast to the response seen in the neuromuscular junction, ethanol markedly decreases acetylcholine release in the brain tissue (following an initial slight increase). This inhibition of acetylcholine release is inversely correlated with endogenous acetylcholine concentrations and it has also been observed in response to the administration of other CNS depressants such as general anaesthetics and barbiturates. This ethanol-induced inhibition of acetylcholine release is much greater than a similar inhibition in the release of dopamine, norepinephrine, serotonin, glutamate and GABA. Ethanol initially increases acetylcholine concentrations, particularly in the corpus striatum and brain stem (Massarelli 1979). But this initial increase is followed by a subsequent decrease in the concentration of acetylcholine in these same regions in chronically intoxicated animals.

The mechanisms underlying these effects are obscure. Ethanol increases the activity of choline acetyltransferase (see above, figure 9), but only at lethal concentrations. It has also been shown to increase the rate of choline uptake by the nerve cells, and the net effect of these two opposing mechanisms upon acetylcholine synthesis is unknown. Contradictory findings have been reported for the effect of ethanol upon the activity of the acetylcholine-degrading enzyme, acetylcholinesterase. Low ethanol concentrations generally enhance acetylcholinesterase activity, whereas larger doses inhibit it; however, some studies have shown that this activity is depressed by even low concentrations of ethanol. Acetyl co-A and coenzyme A concentrations are apparently unaffected by ethanol. These conflicting data make any attempt to interpret the mechanisms underlying the biphasic effect of ethanol upon acetylcholine activity very difficult. However, Massarelli (1979) has suggested a possible model to explain the effects of chronic ethanol intake upon these systems. Ethanol, by packing into the lipid portion of neural membrane systems, alters the charge distributions of those membranes, thus interfering with the ion-dependent processes associated with them and thereby:

(1) affecting choline uptake release, and reuptake across the presynaptic membrane of the axon terminal;[49]

(2) possibly altering the activity of choline acetyltransferase, which is partly bound to the membrane and which is very dependent upon the ionic state of the medium;

(3) altering the response of the different types of postsynaptic receptors with differing affinities for acetylcholine presumed to exist in the neuromuscular junction and in the brain, inasmuch as the receptors themselves are also affected by ionic permeabilities of the postsynaptic membrane;

(4) the enhanced release of acetylcholine at neuromuscular junctions in response to ethanol as contrasted with its reduced release in nervous tissue may partly result from the fact that the acetylcholine precursor, acetyl co-A, is generated primarily from pyruvate in nervous tissue, whereas acetate is the major precursor for acetyl co-A synthesis at the neuromuscular junctions. The high concentrations of acetate resulting from the metabolism of ethanol may cause the enhanced production of acetylcholine at those junctions as compared with the opposite effect induced by ethanol in the peripheral ganglia and the CNS. Finally, acute doses of ethanol may have a general inhibiting effect upon the firing rates of presynaptic, cholinergic neurons which could cause a buildup of acetylcholine in those terminals. This might explain the initial increase

---

[49]Choline reuptake from the synaptic cleft occurs when acetylcholine is broken down into its acetyl co-A and choline moieties by acetylcholinesterase.

in acetylcholine concentrations brought about by ethanol. Chronic insult to neural tissues by ethanol, on the other hand, may alter the membrane-associated, ion-dependent metabolism of choline, thus impairing the long-term synthesis and release of acetylcholine. See also the discussion above on membrane fluidization and increased fusion of synaptic vesicles with the presynaptic membrane; this increases the amount of transmitter released.

The effects of ethanol upon other neurotransmitter systems is more equivocal and the research findings are inconsistent. Acute ethanol challenges have been variously shown to increase, decrease, and have no effect upon the concentration and activity of serotonin. However, ethanol has unequivocally been shown to induce a shift in the peripheral metabolism of serotonin from the oxidative pathway leading to the generation of 5-hydroxyindoleacetate (5-HIAA, see figures 9C and 26) to the reductive pathway which leads to 5-hydroxytryptophol (see also the discussion on condensation products of amines with aldehydes, pages 102–109). Acute doses of ethanol appear to have no effect upon tryptophan hydroxylase (which catalyzes the first step in the synthesis of serotonin, see figure 9C) in the brain, although chronic administration of ethanol increases the activity of this enzyme.

Similarly, work on another inhibitory neurotransmitter, GABA, has also shown increases, decreases, and no change in activity in response to both acute and chronic ethanol (Berry & Pentreath 1980). However, some of this discrepancy may result from the general biphasic effects exerted by ethanol on neurotransmitters and membrane systems. Thus, low doses of ethanol appear to slightly elevate GABA levels in the cerebellum and brain stem, larger doses reduce the GABA levels, and lethal doses produce a marked increase. GABA does appear to potentiate the effects of alcohol intoxication, primarily by enhancing the CNS depressant effects of ethanol. GABA antagonizes the stimulatory effects of low doses of alcohol and compounds the depressant action (recall that alcohol in low doses is stimulatory, with larger doses overriding the initial stimulatory effect). GABA inhibits the action potential at axon terminals by means of axo-axonal junctions similar to those which mediate enkephalin inhibition of synaptic transmission. GABA exerts its major effect upon dopaminergic neurons, inhibiting the release of that neurotransmitter. This inhibitory release appears to be correlated with an accumulation of DA in the brain, perhaps because of an increase in DA synthesis along with the GABA-mediated inhibition of DA release (Berry & Pentreath 1980). The complex interaction between ethanol, GABA and GABA-mediated CNS inhibition is very poorly understood at present, although the overall effect of alcohol administration appears to be to enhance the effects of GABA.

Ethanol enhances the rate of norepinephrine depletion in the brain, but not that of dopamine (which tends to accumulate, as we have just seen), and it has been suggested that ethanol may function as a specific activator of noradrenergic neurons (Noble & Tewari 1978). A single dose of ethanol will increase NE turnover in the brains of rats during the first few hours following administration of the drug. After that time, however, the turnover rates of both NE and DA are reduced. This is compatible with the known biphasic effects of alcohol within the CNS and may explain some of the contradictory findings in the literature. The general effect of ethanol upon neurological systems seems to be one of initial stimulation and subsequent depression. There is some evidence that ethanol noncompetetively inhibits NE presynaptic reuptake, but apparently only at superlethal concentrations (1000 milligrams-percent!).

Alcohol and Vitamin A

The movement of the eyeball is under the control of six striated (skeletal),[50] extraocular muscles, and during visual *fixation* the image of the object under view is directed to the region of the retina with the greatest visual acuity. In normal binocular or stereoscopic vision, the axes of both eyes converge upon the object being viewed because of the action of preconscious reflexes. Acute intoxication by alcohol or other CNS depressants often leads to muscular fatigue and/or loss of coordination between the two eyeballs, and double vision or *diplopia* commonly results. Alcohol-induced diplopia can generally be partially overcome by closing one eye.

The photoreceptive *rods*[51] of the dark-adapted human eye contain a

---

[50]Skeletal muscle, in contrast to smooth muscle such as occurs around the gut, is under voluntary control.

[51]The human retina contains about 60 million rods and 3.5 million cones in each eye (Bowman & Rand 1980). The cones function in bright daylight and are involved in color perception (*photopic vision*), responding selectively to various wavelengths of visible light in the range of 380–780 nannometers (10^{-9} meters from crest to crest). The rods function only in very dim light and they do not respond selectively to various wavelengths; they thus generate only shades of gray (*scotopic vision*). The rods are completely blind in daylight due to the absence of rhodopsin, but slowly become dark-adapted as visual purple accumulates under dark conditions.

pigment called *visual purple* or *rhodopsin* made up of the protein *opsin* conjugated to an aldehyde, *11*-cis-*retinal*—an isomer exhibiting the "boat" configuration at the number 11 carbon (see figure 28). A photon of light impinging upon this system will split the conjugated group into its opsin and retinal moieties and convert the 11-*cis*-retinal into its isomer, *all*-trans-*retinal*—exhibiting an all-"chair" configuration at the number 11 carbon. All-*trans*-retinal is also known as *retinene* and *vitamin A aldehyde*.[52] Meanwhile, a nervous impulse has been sent out via the bipolar cells and second-order neurons to the optic nerve for transmission to the brain.[53] In the absence of light stimulation, all-*trans*-retinal is converted back into 11-*cis*-retinal by an *isomerase*. The 11-*cis*-retinal again combines with opsin, reforming rhodopsin ready once again to capture light energy and repeat the process. In the presence of bright light, both isomers of retinal are reduced to their respective alcohols (*retinol*) by alcohol dehydrogenase, accompanied by the oxidation of NADH into NAD^+. As dark-adaptation proceeds once again in dim light, the two isomers of retinol are converted back into their respective aldehydes and become again available for photoreception. Ethanol is a competetive substrate for alcohol dehydrogenase and in large concentrations it inhibits the formation of retinal from retinol. Night-blindness, the first sign of avitaminosis A, is a common result among alcohol abusers. The conversion of vitamin A (retinol) to retinal is also essential for the normal development of sperm cells, and the competetive inhibition of alcohol dehydrogenase in the testes by ethanol results in testicular atrophy and commonly contributes to sterility and impotence in male alcoholics.

Alcohol, Learning, and Memory

Both acute and chronic ethanol administration appear to decrease the capacity of the brain to synthesize proteins (Noble & Tewari 1978). This decrease appears to be due to (1) inhibition of *aminoacyl-tRNA synthetase*

---

[52]All-*trans*-retinol is also called *vitamin A₁* or *vitamin A alcohol.* This fat-soluble vitamin is readily transported back and forth between the retina and the blood where it is complexed with a retinol-binding carrier protein. It is stored in the liver in large amounts and vitamin A deficiency is rare in developed countries except among certain food faddists and in persons with impaired lipid absorption. Cirrhosis of the liver impairs vitamin A storage and rapid depletion of the body's stores may result in vitamin A deficiency as described above.

[53]A single photon is sufficient to stimulate a potential in a single rod. But because several rods are connected to a single bipolar cell, a minimum of 3 quanta of light (photons) are required to send an impulse on to the optic nerve.

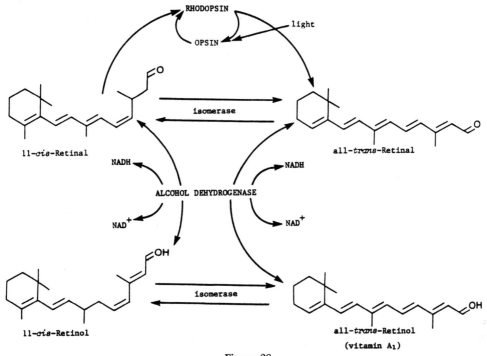

Figure 28
Retinal and Retinol Interactions

activity[54] and (2) disruption of *polyribosomal* function.[55] The significant inhibition of brain protein synthesis resulting from prolonged ethanol challenge occurs both *in vitro* and *in vivo* (Noble & Tewari 1978). This inhibition of brain protein synthesis is associated with a decrease in the amount and activity of transfer RNA and ribosomal RNA. Inside the neuronal nucleus, mRNA responds to an ethanol challenge with an

---

[54]See above, footnote 1 and text, page 3. One transfer RNA exists for each of the 20 amino acids that are incorporated into protein chains linked together by peptide bonds. Each specific tRNA is "charged" with its specific amino acid. Because nucleic acids have no specific affinity for specific amino acids, the recognition and charging of specific amino acids to their specific tRNA molecules is catalyzed by enzymes known as aminoacyl-tRNA-synthetases. There is one specific acyl-tRNA-synthetase for each of the 20 amino acids and their corresponding tRNA molecules. The enzyme removes the hydroxyl group from the carbonyl (−COOH) moiety of the amino acid and attaches to the acyl residue in a process in which ATP is dephosphorylated into adenosine monophosphate (AMP), thus forming an enzyme-AMP-amino acid complex. [An *acyl* is a radical derived from an organic acid by removal of the −OH group.] This complex then recognizes a specific tRNA molecule and transfers the amino acid acyl radical to it. The amino acid remains attached to its tRNA until it is polymerized into a growing protein chain by the ribosomal-mRNA synthesizing factories. See also Light, in press, Volume 4.

[55]Polyribosomes are groups of ribosomes attached to a single mRNA strand during transcription and protein synthesis.

initial increased incorporation of radioactively labelled precursor, followed by a later, very marked depression of such incorporation. This biphasic effect is not seen in cytoplasmic RNA, and it does not appear to involve any alteration in the availability of precursor nucleotides. It is associated with an inhibition in the synthesis of *polyadenylate (polyadenylic acid)*[56] in the brains of animals challenged with ethanol. This system is thought to be involved in the transfer of nuclear mRNA into the cytoplasm and its conversion into the shorter molecules of cytoplasmic mRNA (Noble & Tewari 1978). The decrease in protein synthesis in the brain contrasts markedly with the significant increase in such synthesis in the liver. The latter is associated with the proliferation of the endoplasmic reticulum and Golgi apparatus induced by chronic ethanol intake.

These changes in CNS protein synthesis may have a significant impact upon learning and memory—especially long-term memory. Memory can be categorized into three major processes: (1) *immediate memory*—the registration and storage of information for only a few seconds; (2) *short-term memory*—the transfer of information from immediate memory into a second memory pool where it persists for several minutes or hours; short-term memory involves portions of the thalamus, and in particular the selective attention mechanism which focuses the intensity with which incoming information is assessed and routed into the short-term pool; it appears to be mediated by electrophysiological activity in the neurons involved; (3) *long-term memory*—the consolidation and more or less permanent storage of information and experience transferred from the short-term memory; the formation of long-term memory involves physical changes in the brain which include structural changes in mRNA and the polypeptides and proteins synthesized by that mRNA. Commitment of information to long-term memory may require days or even weeks and the information is stored generally throughout the cerebral cortex, rather than being confined to specific brain regions as are short-term memory processes.

The dendrites of brain cells tend to send out numerous, spontaneous "buds"—the so-called *dendritic spines* which form random synaptic "con-

---

[56]In contrast to the shorter strands of cytoplasmic mRNA (about 2,000 nucleotides), nuclear RNA is much longer and is often referred to as *heterogeneous nuclear RNA*. Both cytoplasmic mRNA and nuclear RNA molecules are capped at their 3'-termini by polyadenylate sequences some 100 to 200 residues in length. The role of such polyadenylate is unclear, but these sequences are added to the nuclear RNA after its transcription from DNA has occurred, and they may be involved in the fragmentation of nRNA into smaller mRNA chains and the transportation of the latter from the nucleus into the cytoplasm where they act in concert with charged tRNA and the ribosomes to synthesize protein molecules.

nections" with nearby axons. These temporary synapses are continuously forming, disintegrating, and reforming, and when present they are available to propagate and anaylze incoming signals. Those synapses which by chance happen to be involved in the transmission and recording of an incoming event tend to become more durable and they do not break down as readily as do those which have not been so engaged. As these more durable pathways are utilized several times in the processing of the information, they become even more permanent and form part of the structural changes that occur in the long-term storage of the information. What began as a simple series of impulse transmission involving only short-term electrical (action potential) and chemical (neurotransmitter release) changes has now become a series of distinct, structural and physical changes in the brain microarchitecture.

Although nuclear DNA is unalterable except by genetic mutation, mRNA can readily be altered by changes in the cellular environment. Chemicals and drugs of various kinds can change the amount and type of proteins synthesized from a given strand of mRNA. Learning has been demonstrated in laboratory animals to be associated with increases in the concentration of nuclear RNA and with changes in the RNA base-pair ratios (the relative proportion of adenosine appears to increase over that of uracil). The CNS of all animals tested thus far (including mammals, birds and reptiles) contains a specific protein found only in the brain. This protein is known as *S-100* and it has exactly the same amino acid sequence in all taxa; S-100 antiserum cross-reacts in all species. It is found in glial cell bodies and in the nuclei of neurons. It binds to Ca^{2+} and can undergo conformational changes as a result of the redistribution of its ionic charges. Training in laboratory rats causes an increase in the total amount of S-100 in the cells of the hippocampus. Furthermore, such training also produces an extra electrophoretic band[57] containing a higher than normal level of Ca^{2+}. These changes in S-100 that result from learning are not permanent, however, and they do not even persist throughout the duration of the animals' performance. This lack of persistence on the part of S-100 has two possible explanations (Seiden & Dykstra 1977): (1) it may be merely an intermediate molecule which induces the formation of still another molecule; (2) and perhaps more likely, the S-100 may become absorbed into the cell membrane where it

---

[57]Electrophoresis is the separation of the differently charged components of proteins in an electric field; each specific protein exhibits its own unique signature.

escapes detection. Despite the temporary nature of S-100 in the learning process, its experimental destruction also causes the destruction of memory, and the administration of S-100 antiserum also disrupts the acquisition of information. Learning in mice is associated with increased production of nuclear RNA, as well as of ribosomal and polysomal RNA.

The suggestion that protein synthesis plays an important role in learning is supported by studies in which RNA and polypeptides taken from trained planarian worms and laboratory rodents and injected into untrained animals facilitate the acquisition of the same training in the latter. Furthermore, the administration of antibiotics which inhibit specific phases of protein synthesis can cause impairment in both short-term and long-term memory. Thus, the implications of CNS protein synthesis reduction due to both acute and chronic ethanol insult for learning and memory impairment seem clear.

Some agents facilitate learning and memory. Strychnine and amphetamines both enhance neural transmission, the former by blocking central inhibitory neurotransmitters and the latter by enhancing the action of dopamine and norepinephrine. Antidiuretic hormone or vasopressin (see Light 1985 for a discussion of this) is also known to enhance learning and memory function. Alcohol inhibits the release of vasopressin from the hypothalamus and this may perhaps play a role in alcohol-induced memory deficits. However, caffeine and theophylline also block vasopressin release, yet learning appears to be facilitated by these drugs; it may be that learning enhancement because of general CNS stimulation overshadows any decrement due to lack of vasopressin. And, of course, these influences may be so slight that their effects are insignificant relative to other factors.

Degenerative changes in the thalamus, mammillary bodies and hippocampus brought about by long-term alcohol abuse are involved in the etiology of Wernicke-Korsakoff psychosis. The destruction of the hippocampus on only one side results in minor memory deficits. Left hippocampal lesions give rise to verbal impairment, whereas damage to the right hippacampus causes loss of ability to remember new faces, shapes or musical phrases. Destruction of both hippocampi cause drastic impairment which are greater than the sums of the deficits produced by destruction of only one side or the other (Calvin & Ojemann 1980). Such bilateral hippacampal lesions prevent the short-term memory from retaining new information long enough for it to be committed to the long-term memory. Both the immediate and long-term memories remain intact and the individual can recall events that occurred only a few minutes before or long-term events that took place years ago, before the hippocampal damage had occurred.

Wernicke-Korsakoff's syndrome in addition to the type of hippocampal destruction just described, also involves lesions in the thalamus and mammillary bodies. The thalamic lesions impair the normal operation of the selective attention mechanism and further prevent the retention of new information for a sufficient length of time for it to be committed to long-term memory. The lesions in the mammillary bodies produce an apathetic, docile individual who typically exhibits a previous history of aggression and violence.[58]

Korsakoff's-stage syndrome is characterized by disorientation, confusion, both anterograde and retrograde amnesia (although the former is predominant), and confabulation. The patient is typically alert and responsive and the consciousness is not clouded. Korsakoff's syndrome typically arises following one or more episodes of Wernicke's syndrome in which clouding of the sensorium is a prominent feature, or it may develop without any previous involvement of Wernicke's signs. Like many other neurological disorders associated with chronic alcohol abuse, Wernicke-Korsakoff's syndrome has traditionally been attributed to malnutrition—especially thiamine deficiency. However, several nutritionally-controlled studies (Freund 1976; Butters & Cermak 1980) have conclusively shown that, although thiamine and other deficiencies are frequently involved, most of the neuropathological consequences of ethanol abuse derive from the direct, cytotoxic effects of alcohol upon nervous tissue. True Korsakoff's syndrome cannot be preduced by even severe thiamine and other nutritional deficiencies acting alone; chronic and severe alcohol intake is a necessary concomitant.

A series of studies in which alcohol was given to laboratory animals along with a nutritionally adequate diet have demonstrated learning impairment following 3–7 months of chronic ethanol consumption (Walker *et al.* 1980). This impairment did not remit even after the animals had been ethanol-free for 18 weeks! Retention of an acquired task is also impaired regardless of whether the prolonged ethanol consumption precedes or follows the learning event (Freund 1976), perhaps due to altered CNS protein metabolism. Interestingly, chronic phenobarbital

---

[58]The mammillary bodies are involved in the expression of rage and aggression, and they are normally under the inhibitory control of the amygdala (see above, page 56).

sedation does not result in such learning or retention impairment. In a series of follow-up studies, Walker *et al.* (1980) demonstrated ethanol-produced alterations in dendrite morphology and the number of neurons within the hippocampus and cerebellum after several months of chronic ethanol intake along with a nutritionally adequate diet. The number of dendritic spines on hippocampal and cerebellar neurons was significantly lower than in controls (by 50–60% P < 0.001).[59] the degree of dendritic branching in the cerebellar *Purkinje cells*[60] is significantly reduced relative to controls (P < 0.05). In addition, hippocampal and cerebellar neurons in alcohol-treated rats showed a number of abnormal Golgi bodies (which are involved in the export of proteins). These abnormalities are produced in the hippocampus and cerebellum of ethanol-treated rats, but such lesions do not apparently arise in the thalamus or in the caudate nucleus. It is not clear whether these changes are due to degenerative processes in the affected neurons themselves or because of transynaptic degeneration associated with the loss of afferent synaptic input. Furthermore, rats treated with ethanol for five months exhibit 16 percent fewer hippocampal and cerebellar cells, along with the presence of numerous, dark-staining bodies in many of the remaining cells. These bodies are very much like those produced by vascular interruption and its consequent hypoxia in those same tissues (Walker *et al.* 1980).

Recently, computerized axial tomography (CAT) scans of the brains of chronic alcoholics have revealed major differences in the densities and total mass of tissue in the cerebral cortex relative to normal controls. The volume shrinkage is revealed by widening of the sulci (the valleys between the ridges or gyri) and Sylvian fissure (the deep fissure separating the temporal and parietal lobes). Ventricular enlargement[61] is also a prominent feature in the brains of alcoholics. These brain changes are established quite early in the drinking careers of alcoholic patients and they

---

[59]This figure is the probability associated with the null hypothesis that the measurements of the ethanol-treated rats are not different from those of the untreated rats, *i.e.*, that the administration of alcohol has no effect. The probability values calculated from the data of these experiments state that the chances that the observed deviations (of the treated animals) are due strictly to chance alone are less than 0.1%. In other words, the investigators are more than 99.9% sure that the deviations are due to the effects of ethanol treatment.

[60]Large branching cells in the middle layer of the cerebellar cortex; these cells are inhibitory and prevent the kind of reverberatory activity seen in the R.A.S. and the cerebral cortex.

[61]The remnants of the spaces formed by the hollow tube of the developing brain and spinal cord (the two lateral ventricles, the diencephalon and the 4th ventricle).

do not appear to be correlated with the severity or length of drinking (Lishman *et al.* 1980). Young alcoholics exhibit the same brain pathologies as do older ones, although there are very minor differences in the extent of the damage that do correlate with age. Only minor improvement in these degenerative brain changes have been observed after prolonged abstinence (one year or more), although the long-term prognosis is unknown.

More recently, direct evidence of decreased brain densities have been reported (Golden *et al.* 1981). In a study of young chronic alcoholics (nine males and two females in both the alcoholic and control groups) with an average age of 29.36 ± 6.4 years and a mean drinking career of 8.27 ± 5.62 years, significant differences were found in the densities of their brains relative to the controls. In addition, there was significantly more degeneration and ventricle enlargement in the left cerebral hemisphere of the alcoholic group than in the right hemisphere. In the control group only 2 out of 33 measurements was the right hemisphere more dense than the left, and both of those measurements came from the same individual. In the alcoholic group, on the other hand, 10 out of 33 comparisons showed denser right cerebral hemispheres. It should be pointed out that both the alcoholic and control groups were carefully screened for any history of neurological deficit or seizure activity. The data suggest a deficit in the density of the left hemisphere in young chronic alcoholics, whereas no such deficit was demonstrated for the right hemisphere. The left cerebral hemisphere appears to be physiologically more susceptible to the toxic effects of chronic ethanol abuse. Because psychological testing of alcoholics has consistently shown impairment of nonverbal functions, it has been assumed that the primary lesions were in the right hemisphere known to be involved in those functions (Golden *et al.* 1981). The authors point out, however, that the left hemisphere plays a strong role in non-verbal processes, and that verbal functions are strongly overlearned in any case, and very resistant to the ravages of slowly developing disorders such as alcoholism.

The clinical manifestations of cerebellar degeneration include gradual development of ataxia, incoordination, spasticity, gross tremors of the limbs, nystagmus and thick speech. *Marchiafava-Bignami disease* is a rare disorder that may be uniquely precipitated by alcoholism. It is characterized by degeneration of the corpus callosum, which consists primarily of myelinated fibers connecting the two cerebral hemispheres, and an insidious onset of manic, depressive or paranoid psychosis along with a number of other neurological signs, including dementia, grand mal seizures, mild paralysis, inability to initiate voluntary movements, and loss of speech. Death commonly occurs within three to six years after the onset of this disorder (Freund 1976).

Chronic ethanol administration in rats produces intrinsic changes in the phospholipid to protein ratio in the membrane component of myelin sheaths from the brain stem. The phospholipid portion is reduced by about 20% in rats given oral ethanol doses for one year. Cholesterol to protein ratios are also reduced by chronic ethanol administration, and these changes are reflective of a degenerative change in myelin. This degenerative change is not the same as the adaptive changes exhibited by neuronal membranes in the development of tolerance to the effects of chronic alcohol challenge. The adaptive changes of neuronal membranes is largely reversible upon cessation of alcohol intake, whereas the reduction in phospholipid and cholesteral is largely irreversible in myelin because it lacks the necessary enzymes to rebuild and maintain the membrane system. The decrease in myelin phospholipid content may be due to the activation of degradative phospholipases in the cellular portions of myelin sheaths. Cerebral degeneration is most closely associated with those brain regions rich in myelin material. Myelin cholesterol appears to be less susceptible to alcohol-induced reduction than are phospholipids. As with any such study using animal models for human responses to alcohol, the results, although strongly suggestive, must be interpreted with caution. There are many species-specific differences in the response to drugs and the features exhibited by rats do not always apply to mice or cats, let alone to humans.

The denegerative changes seen in the brains of chronic alcoholics are similar to those associated with aging, and several authors have suggested that chronic alcohol abuse accelerates the aging process (Freund 1976; Walker *et al.* 1980). Interestingly, tetrahydro-beta-carboline condensates (see above) accumulate in the lens of the human eye as a function of increasing age. Mental decline associated with aging ranges from slightly increased forgetfulness to profound senility and dementia, often with florid paranoid psychoses. The more severe deterioration associated with aging has generally been ascribed to *Alzheimer's disease* and attributed to the loss of a critical number of cortical neurons. Similar hippocampal lesions have been noted in both senile and alcoholic laboratory animals. However, as Freund (1976) has observed, a great number of diverse disorders can produce similar neurological lesions and result in similar functional impairment. Furthermore, Alzheimer's disease has recently (Kolata 1983) been associated with specific degenerative changes in the cholinergic neurons whose cell bodies are located in the *nucleus basalis* located in the basal forebrain right above the optic chiasma. The axons of these neurons project to all parts of the cerebral cortex, and as these neurons fail, degenerative plaques begin to form in the cortex in the vicinity of their axons. The plaques may form in response to the reduced levels of acetylcholine which may prevent the cortical neurons from functioning properly. It may be that the decline in brain function associated with aging is due to a wide range of factors, including genetic predisposition, previous illness complicated by neuronal death, and chronic toxic insult such as lifelong alcohol abuse.

The neurological consequences of hepatic encephalopathy were reviewed in Volume 1 of this series (Light 1985). The primary toxic mechanism appears to be ammonia buildup in the brain because of the failure of hepatic detoxification mechanisms. A number of nonspecific personality and intellectual changes may occur, and the course may range from deep coma and death to variable improvement or progressive deterioration over several years.

Peripheral polyneuropathy or disorders of the peripheral nervous system may arise in the motor, sensory and autonomic systems in response to a variety of ethanol-related causes.[62] Signs and symptoms can range from asymptomatic to severe neurological pathology and disability. Most chronic alcoholics exhibit no detectable peripheral nervous impairment but peripheral neuropathy does occur in 5–15% of alcoholics (Schuckit 1979). When peripheral polyneuropathy does occur, its progression is generally slow and progresses over a period of weeks or months. The impairment is typically bilateral, affecting both sides of the body and it commences and is generally more severe in the lower body and distal rather than in the upper and proximal extremities. Numbness, pain, hypersensitivity to pressure accompanied by muscular weakness and atrophy, foot and wrist drop and ataxia are common manifestations of peripheral neurological impairment resulting from chronic alcohol abuse. Autonomic nervous system functions may also become impaired and give rise to vocal cord disorders manifested by chronic hoarseness and vocal weakness, chronic hypotension and a variety of other difficulties. In very

[62]This review is from Freund (1976).

severe cases the cranial nerves themselves may become involved and deficits in visual field and other ocular impairment and paralysis of the muscles of the face, eyes and pharynx may be the result.

There is no question that much of this polyneuropathy is produced by the direct, cytotoxic effect of ethanol upon neural tissues such as was previously described. However, severe deficiencies in vitamins B are also involved in these disorders and adequate vitamin therapies can improve many cases of alcoholic peripheral polyneuropathy if the damage has not progressed beyond the point of recovery. Most investigators agree that ethanol-associated polyneuropathies cannot be generated by avitaminosis B alone, and that the neuropathologies due solely to vitamin deficiency is clinically different from those seen in chronic alcoholics. Furthermore, many alcoholics do manifest polyneuropathies in the absence of vitamin deficiency or malnutrition. Demyelination of the axons associated with vitamin deficiency occurs only in the last stages, whereas primary axonal degeneration commonly occurs in the early stages of alcoholic polyneuropathy.

Sleep, Rebound Phenomena, and Alcohol Withdrawal

The interaction of the raphe nuclei, locus coeruleus and the R.A.S. and the relative activities of neurotransmitter substances in the sleep-wake cycle have been briefly described (see above). Normal sleep consists of two phases: REM sleep and non-REM sleep. These two phases of sleep together with wakefulness have been referred to as the three "states of consciousness" (Mendelson 1979). The waking state is characterized by an EEG[63] pattern of low-voltage, mixed frequency waves. When the eyes are closed and in a relaxed state prior to entering sleep, the pattern shifts to the regular rhythm characteristic of *alpha-waves*. Non-REM sleep commences as stage 1, light-sleep, and the brain waves diminish in amplitude and frequency (4–6 Hz or cycles/second). Stage 2 non-REM sleep is characterized by more irregular and even slower waves of larger amplitude interspersed with brief, rapid bursts of *sleep spindles* and *K-complexes;* the latter consist of a small, sharp wave followed by one or two larger waves and a series of fast waves of 12 Hz, and they arise in response to specific, significant stimuli such as the cry of one's child or sound of one's own name. Non-REM stages 3 and 4 exhibit increasingly larger-

---

[63]Electroencephalograph.

amplitude and slower frequency (1–2 Hz) *delta waves,* and are collectively known as *slow-wave sleep* (SWS). Sleep spindles are present during SWS but in stage 4 they are infrequent and K-complexes cannot be elicited, which distinguishes it from stage 3. Stage 4 non-REM sleep is of short duration and occurs only two or three times in the first half or so of the night. It is interrupted by periods of REM sleep exhibiting high-frequency, low-voltage, mixed-frequency waves similar to those of the wakeful state. REM sleep is accompanied by active dreaming along with rapid shifting of the eyeballs and total atonia or relaxation of the major lower-body muscles (see pages 59-61). The first episode of REM sleep occurs from one to two hours after the onset of non-REM sleep. These alternating cycles of REM and non-REM sleep continue throughout the night about every 90 minutes or so in young adults, but stage 4 non-REM sleep disappears completely in the latter half of the night. Likewise, more SWS sleep occurs during the first part of the night, whereas REM sleep predominates towards morning. Normally, REM sleep comprises 25% or so of total sleep time.

Alcohol affects this normal pattern in a variety of ways.[64] Ethanol has a general sedative effect in nonalcoholic human subjects evidenced primarily by a decrease in *sleep latency* or the period of time required to fall asleep after going to bed, rather than any change in total sleep time. Decreased REM sleep is universally observed especially during the first half of the night, and this may occur even when the alcohol was taken several hours prior to sleep and with blood ethanol concentrations of 50 mg-percent or less, well below that associated with overt intoxication. With low to moderate doses of ethanol (3½ ounces) REM sleep is suppressed during the first portion of the night, but actually increased during the second half of the sleep cycle; the increase in percentage of REM sleep during the second half of the night may even "wash out" the decrease observed during the first period, resulting in no net change in REM sleep percentage over the course of the entire night. When higher doses are given (6 ounces), the REM sleep percentage is significantly decreased during both halves of the night. The mechanisms behind this apparent biphasic effect of ethanol upon REM sleep are obscure. When ethanol is chronically administered in the usual clinical doses of approximately 1 gm per kilogram of body weight to nonalcoholic human subjects, the initial decrease in REM sleep percentage returns to baseline (or even slightly above) values by the second or third night. Upon cessation of

---

[64]The following review is taken largely from Mendelson (1979).

ethanol intake a *rebound* increase in REM sleep is commonly observed. Such REM rebound is characteristic of drugs which produce tolerance and dependence.

Alcoholics abstinent for three weeks exhibit more REM and stage 1 non-REM sleep than age-matched controls; they also have less stage 3 non-REM sleep. Younger alcoholics from 24–39 years also show less stage 4 non-REM sleep than age-matched normal subjects—this difference does not occur in older alcoholics presumably due to the normal decrease in stage 4 sleep with increasing age in the normal subjects. The increased REM sleep is associated with shorter REM/non-REM cycles, and the sleep of abstinent alcoholics is also characterized by increases in arousal and changes of sleep cycles than is seen in normal persons. Such decreased slow-wave sleep and increased frequency of stage changes appears to last for at least one to two years in abstinent alcoholics (Mendelson 1979), and one study suggested that normal slow-wave sleep may not return for nearly four years (Adamson & Burdick 1973 *in* Mendelson 1979). The disturbed sleep and decreased SWS of alcoholics has been compared to the sleep of elderly persons.

When abstinent alcoholics resume drinking there is a decrease in REM sleep percentage often accompanied by an increase in SWS percentage, and ethanol appears to shorten the interval between REM sleep episodes analogous to that observed in normal subjects. Drinking alcoholics tend to sleep in several brief periods and there may be an overall increase in total sleep time over a 24-hour period (Mello & Mendelson 1970 *in* Mendelson 1979).

Upon cessation of alcohol intake alcoholics frequently exhibit a reduction of total sleep time, and after several nights the percentage of REM sleep increases drastically over that of normal subjects, sometimes equalling 90% (!) of total sleep time. This seems to involve an increase in the number of REM sleep episodes and a decrease in the intervals between such episodes. The degree of increase in REM sleep appears to correlate positively with the occurrence of hallucinosis and delerium tremens. A major difference in the REM sleep rebound phenomenon between alcoholics and normal subjects is that the rebound is delayed for a few days upon withdrawal of ethanol in alcoholic persons.

The relationship between depression and alcoholism has been repeatedly stressed in this book. Likewise, the correlation between neurotransmitter imbalances, particularly deficits of norepinephrine and serotonin, and depression has also been emphasized. Alcoholics generally present with "agitated" depression, characterized by often severe insomnia, restlessness, anxiety, irritability, resentment, anger and hostility. They are very prone to explosive emotional outbursts and their general affective complexion is one of chronic dysphoria—particularly during periods of abstinence from alcohol. This type of depression may involve serotonin deficits as a major etiological factor, and many of the symptoms perhaps arise as a result of inhibitory release of the R.A.S., limbic and hypothalamic nuclei involved in arousal, and of emotional experience and expression. Several studies have reported that ethanol exerts a potentiating effect upon serotonin-mediated functions in laboratory animals. Several weeks of ethanol administration results in an increased concentration of brain serotonin in rats (Bowman & Rand 1980). Ethanol alone has no effect upon REM sleep latency whereas the administration of L-tryptophan (the amino acid precursor of serotonin) caused a small but significant decrease in that parameter. When ethanol and L-tryptophan are administered together the decrease in REM sleep latency is greatly potentiated. The mechanism whereby these two agents interact synergistically is not known. The disturbed, abnormal sleep patterns characteristic of abstinent alcoholics may be due to serotoninergic dysfunction as has already been suggested. In this regard, one study reported that the fragmented REM sleep episodes exhibited by dry alcoholics is substantially alleviated by the administration of 5-hydroxy-tryptophan (Zarcone & Hoddes 1975 *in* Mendelson 1979). The study concluded that abnormal sleep due to serotoninergic dysfunction may be persistent in abstinent alcoholics. Serum tryptophan levels increase in rodents up to four hours following an ethanol challenge and decreases occur later at about seven hours (Lieber 1982). And most studies show that brain levels of both serotonin and its major metabolite, 5-HIAA or 5-hydroxyindoleacetic acid, are elevated following alcohol administration. Significantly, cerebrospinal fluid levels are increased in alcoholics during intoxication and decreased during abstinence.

It was recently reported (Naranjo *et al.* 1984) that regular doses of *zimelidine*, an antidepressant approved in Europe but not in the United States, caused heavy social drinkers (subjects not regarded as "alcoholic," but who normally drink at least 28 drinks per week) to significantly reduce their drinking. These subjects, who presented no symptoms of physical or psychiatric problems, typically reduced their drinking by 15–20% by the second day of receiving zimelidine, as compared to placebo which elicited no such change in drinking activity. These subjects returned to previous levels of ethanol intake by the second day after zimelidine was discontinued. All the subjects scored low on anxiety and depression tests both prior to and following the treatment. Very noteworthy, however, in view of the suggested relationship between serotonin insufficiency, depression, and alcoholism, zimelidine acts specifically by inhibiting presynaptic serotonin reuptake!

Both rats and hamsters kept in prolonged darkness drink significantly more ethanol than they do when maintained in photoperiods of alternating light and darkness. Rats kept in constant darkness exhibit much larger pineal bodies than do animals maintained in illumination. Darkness is also known to enhance the activity of N-acetyltransferase and hydroxyindole-O-methyltransferase [= N-acetyl-serotonin-O-methyltransferase], enzymes which catalyze the conversion of serotonin to melatonin in the pineal body (see above). Melatonin levels are highest at night, and deficiencies of this substance due to low levels of its precursor, serotonin, may exacerbate the effects of insomnia. It has been suggested that prolonged darkness enhances the conversion of serotonin to melatonin, causing a depletion of the former, and that this induced serotonin deficit is associated with the development of a preference for increased ethanol intake in rats and hamsters (Geller & Purdy 1979). The implication is that decreased brain levels of serotonin may induce a preference for ethanol whereas increased brain serotonin concentrations would be expected to decrease ethanol preference. Rats given 5-hydroxytryptophan do show such a decrease in ethanol preference relative to controls, as do animals administered serotonin intraventricularly. Moreover, a serotonin antagonist, *cinanserin*, which operates through receptor blockade, also increases ethanol intake. All these data give compelling support to the hypothesis that alcoholism involves deficits in the normal function of brain serotoninergic systems, resulting in a chronic dysphoric depression and an increasing need to self-medicate with beverage alcohol.

Serotonin is also found in the islet cells (islets of Langerhans) of the pancreas, where it apparently exerts an inhibitory modulating effect upon insulin release. In view of the association of reactive hypoglycemia with both depression and alcoholism, it is tempting to speculate that imbalances in this neurotransmitter may be involved in the chronic glucose intolerance seen in these populations. However, the actual dynamics of serotoninergic inhibition of insulin release by the islet cells are unknown and such speculation is tenuous at best. Furthermore, brain serotonin deficiency is not necessarily associated with lowered plasma serotonin levels—serotonin is synthesized within the axon terminals of central neurons from tryptophan which is actively transported across the neural membrane by a carrier protein. Serotonin deficits in the CNS may or may not be correlated with similar deficits in the islets of Langerhans.

The *ethanol-withdrawal syndrome* or *abstinence syndrome* is divided into three phases of increasing severity:

(1) *First phase withdrawal*—indicative of mild to moderate dependence. The onset of first phase withdrawal symptoms and signs occurs within 8 to 24 hours after cessation of drinking and after the ethanol has been completely cleared from the body. It is characterized by psychomotor agitation and tremors, anxiety and apprehension, muscular weakness, nausea, often with retching, and anorexia. These responses are immediately controlled by ethanol and this may lead to matutinal (morning) drinking.

(2) *Second phase withdrawal*—indicative of moderate to severe dependence. With continued abstinence from ethanol and after 12 to 24 hours of first phase withdrawal, severe tremor, muscle cramps, sweating and a rise in body temperature, diarrhea, severe nausea and vomiting, tachycardia and elevated blood pressure, and hyperventillation accompanied by a dramatic change over from metabolic acidosis to respiratory alkalosis (see Light 1985) predominate. There is severe insomnia with only brief, fitful intervals of pure REM sleep characterized by nightmares and extreme agitation.

(3) *Third phase withdrawal*—delirium tremens, indicative of extreme physical dependence. This florid and life-threatening syndrome typically begins 2 to 4 days after the cessation of drinking and the signs and symptoms of phases 1 and 2 are continued into this phase. Delirium tremens is characterized by confusion and disorientation, extreme agitation and panic, delusions, and marked paranoid hallucinations, the latter typically auditory and frequently preceded by unusual sensitivity to sounds, although tactile and usually (but not always) terrifying visual hallucinations are also common. The tremor seen in the earlier abstinence phases become gross shakes accompanied by muscular spasms and jerks. Petit mal seizures may occur, these commonly progressing to grand mal seizures and even *status epilepticus*, a dangerous, life-threatening state of continuous grand mal seizures with no intervening period of recovery. The mortality rate in fulminant and untreated cases of delirium tremens varies from 15% to more

than 50% (Bowman & Rand 1980). In the absence of treatment this phase may last for three to four days, and it terminates in a deep sleep from which the patient emerges clear and lucid.

The signs and symptoms of ethanol withdrawal have been referred to several different CNS disturbances approximately correlated with the severity of the withdrawal (Feuerlein 1980). *Factor 1 Reactions* derive from dysfunctions of cortical and sensory pathways and include: nausea, vomiting, tinnitus (ringing of the ear), visual and sleep disturbances, agitation, and tactile, visual and/or auditory hallucinations. *Factor 2 Reactions* derive from affective disturbances of the limbic system and are thought to include: tremor, paroxysmal sweats, depression and anxiety. *Factor 3 Reactions* are thought to derive from disturbances in brain stem function, including the cerebellum, and include: impairment of consciousness and reality contact, clouding of the sensorium (loss of mental clarity accompanied by confusion and disorientation), gait disturbances (ataxia) and nystagmus. Factors 1 and 2 are known to occur while ethanol is still being ingested and these responses are exacerbated when ethanol is withdrawn. Factor 3 responses are also known to occur while blood ethanol levels are greater than zero.

There is extreme individual variability in the clinical manifestations of ethanol withdrawal responses. Most patients exhibit only minor signs and symptoms characteristic of first phase withdrawal syndrome. However, others who cannot be clinically distinguished from the former may progress into second and third phase reactions. Becker *et al.* (1974) have divided the spectrum of alcoholic abstinence syndrome into two major categories (see figure 29)—*minor* and *major*. Minor withdrawal reactions typically occur within eight hours or so following the last drink,[65] and are characterized for the most part by gross tremors. This initial response is quickly alleviated by further alcohol intake. According to Becker *et al.* (1974), alcoholic hallucinosis and withdrawal seizures generally occur within 24 hours following the cessation of alcohol intake and they are rare after 36 hours of abstinence. On the other hand, alcoholic hallucinations frequently become even more severe at this point along with exacerbated signs of autonomic involvement, including agitation, increased

---

[65]The abstinence syndrome depends more upon the rate of fall of blood alcohol levels than upon absolute blood concentrations *per se*, and the last drink may not indicate the actual onset of the withdrawal response. Conversely, even minor withdrawal manifestations may first occur three to four days after hospitalization (Becker *et al.* 1974).

pulse, sweating and fever and even more severe shakes. The earlier hallucinations tend to occur with a clear and unclouded sensorium and the patient is often clear about the hallucinatory nature of his experience. Persistent hallucinatory activity tends to co-occur with increased agitation and is associated with disorientation and a severely clouded consciousness typical of delirium tremens. Becker *et al.* (1974) report that the hallucinosis associated with delirium tremens is by no means always of a frightening nature to their patients. The minor and major withdrawal states described by these authors merge imperceptibly into each other, and some patients develop an atypical pattern in which a fixed, frequently paranoid, delusional state is paramount. These authors caution that strict criteria with regard to the time of onset and duration of hallucinatory and delusional features should not be employed too stringently in differentiating alcoholic from functional[66] psychoses. Mistakenly administering phenothiazine antipsychotic agents to a deluded or hallucinating alcoholic in severe withdrawal may lower the seizure threshold and needlessly endanger the patient's life.[67] In the experience of these authors (Becker *et al.* 1974), seizures rarely occur after the onset of hallucinations whereas transient hallucinosis and even delirium tremens commonly follow the termination of withdrawal seizures.

Psychological stress appears to potentiate seizure activity during severe alcohol withdrawal, a phenomenon that is well known to staff personnel in hospital detoxification wards. An unnanounced walk through such a ward by a uniformed policeman is often enough to precipitate a seizure in one or more of the inpatients (O'Briant & Lennard 1973). Many nonmedical detox units employ reduced, but constant lighting, piped in music and other soothing stimuli to reduce the incidence of seizures and the severity and frequency of hallucinations. Such stress reactions to the chaotic and alarming environment of alien and white-dominated metropolitan emergency rooms may partially account for the greater frequency of alcoholic hallucinosis among American black males relative to the rest of the population (see Light 1985). Young ghetto blacks typically

---

[66]The *functional psychoses* are distinguished from those resulting from organic brain or other dysfunction, in that the former occur in the absence of any known organic disorder. However, as discussed earlier, several of the "functional" psychoses are now known to be largely due to CNS neurotransmitter dysfunction—for example, schizophrenia and manic-depressive disorder, and this distinction has lost much of its former significance.

[67]Pre-existing seizure disorders can be greatly exacerbated by the ethanol withdrawal event following even a single, moderate drinking episode by a nonalcoholic person, and such persons are probably better advised never to drink beverage alcohol at all.

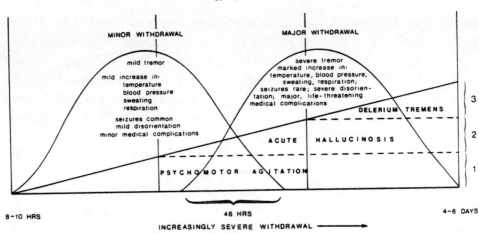

Figure 29

Phases of the Ethanol Withdrawal Syndrome

The two normal curves represent the signs of minor and major withdrawal as described and figured by Becker et al., 1974. The diagonal line running from lower left to upper right represents progressively severe withdrawal. The three elongated horizontal blocks are the major factor reactions proposed by Feurerlein (1979; see above, page 130), and the numbers at the right side of the graph represent the designations used by Feuerlein. Factor 1 reactions derive from cortical and sensory dysfunctions and include: nausea, vomiting, tinnitis, visual and sleep disturbances, agitation, and hallucinations. Factor 2 reactions derive from limbic disturbances and include: tremor, sweating, depression and anxiety. Factor 3 reactions are due to brain stem dysfunction and include: clouding of consciousness, impaired reality contact, confusion, and motor disturbances.

restrict themselves very closely to the narrow confines of their own territory in the inner city, and many of them have little personal experience outside that milieu. The rare occasions in which they do venture outside into the "white" world are typically frightening and overwhelmingly stressful experiences for many of them (Mrs. Carmen Dixon, M.S.W., personal communication, 1976). That the alcoholic withdrawal reactions should suddenly become more severe in such patients in the typical county hospital emergency room setting is hardly surprising in view of the foregoing discussion.

In point of fact, psychological stress is known to potentiate the pharmacological effects of other drugs to a very dangerous extent—even to the point of causing death itself! An elegantly conducted and well-controlled recent study (Siegel *et al.* 1982) has convincingly demonstrated that death from heroin overdose is very largely a function of the anxiety level of the addict. Many experienced heroin addicts die from doses that should not be life-threatening in view of the degree of tolerance of the addict to the drug, and many die from doses that were well tolerated just the day before. Environmental cues associated with the drug-taking behavior are a critical factor in the potentiation of heroin overdose reactions, and many overdose deaths occur when the addict takes either a normally well-tolerated dose or a higher-than-usual dose in an unfamiliar setting. When morphine is injected in the presence of environmental cues different from those previously signalling the drug, both humans and laboratory rats exhibit significantly less tolerance than would otherwise be the case. Physiological and pharmacodynamic tolerance to opiates develops independently of environmental circumstances, but suddenly altering the accustomed setting for drug-taking in a tolerant addict is enough to precipitate a fatal reaction. Rats with the same pharmacological history of heroin administration differ significantly in mortality rates when challenged with a lethal dose, depending upon whether or not the drug is administered in the accustomed or a different setting (in the case of the rats, it was a matter of which cage in which they took the drug). Mortality is significantly greater in those animals challenged with a heroic dose in an environment other than the one in which they were used to receiving the drug. Many replications of these experiments were consistent (Siegel *et al.* 1982). The obvious implications of this study for withdrawal potentiation in addicted human beings seems clear.

It has been suggested (Mendelson 1979; Bowman & Rand 1980) that alcoholic hallucinosis is due to the "intrusions" of dreams associated with the rebound increase in REM sleep spilling over into wakefulness. Such a spillover of dream material into the wakeful state has also been suggested as the primary dynamic behind schizophrenic hallucinations and it is thought to derive from impairment of the selective attention mechanism associated with dopaminergic neurons in the thalamus and corpus striatum. This suggestion has been criticized on the grounds that REM sleep rebounds often occur without hallucinations or nightmares after withdrawal of moderate amounts of alcohol even in nonalcoholic control subjects. Similarly, REM sleep rebound may also occur without psychotic episodes upon withdrawal of many other agents, including Δ^9-tetrahydrocannabinol, the active ingredient in marijuana and hashish. However, this by no means precludes a casual relationship between REM sleep rebound and alcoholic hallucinosis and/or delirium tremens since the actual dynamics of such interactions are almost certainly extremely complex and modified by many other factors. Many alcoholics with extreme physical dependency do not manifest hallucinations or delirium tremens upon abstinence from ethanol although they may present many of the other signs and symptoms of severe withdrawal, including seizures. It has also been observed that the REM sleep rebound effect differs to some degree in alcoholics and normal subjects. Abstinence induced REM sleep rebound in the alcoholic is generally delayed for several days following cessation of drinking, whereas it occurs immediately following such abstinence in normal persons (Mendelson 1979). It has also been suggested that the REM sleep rebound potential of a drug is indicative of its addictive potential. Thus such highly addictive agents as the barbiturates, amphetamines and opiate alkaloids also suppress REM sleep during chronic administration, and this REM sleep depression is typically followed by a rebound increase following withdrawal. Other psychoactive drugs without significant addictive potential, but which also suppress REM sleep during administration—for example chlorpromazine and lithium—generate no such REM sleep rebound upon withdrawal.

Ethanol is known to protect experimental animals against drug and electrically generated convulsions, presumably by raising the seizure threshold. However, a rebound reduction in this threshold commonly occurs following withdrawal of the ethanol. This effect apparently occurs after only one dose and it has been reported in patients being treated for depression with electroconvulsive therapy. This post-withdrawal lowering of the seizure threshold may enhance seizure activity due to a variety of metabolic and nutritional causes (see also footnote 68). Among such factors are electrolyte and water imbalance (and in particular, magnesium deficiency or hypomagnesemia) resulting from long-standing poor nutrition and ethanol-generated lactic acidosis and ketoacidosis (see Light 1985). Likewise, hypoglycemia due to a variety of alcohol-related dysfunctions, can produce grand mal seizures. The magnesium deficiency due to alcoholic acidosis is generally masked by the maintainence of metabolic acidosis resulting from continued ethanol intake. Magnesium loss occurs with marked diuresis, including that produced by the inhibition of vasopressin release due to ethanol's effect upon the posterior pituitary. Hypomagnesemia is also brought about by a variety of malabsorbtion syndromes due to ethanol toxicity (Light 1985) and the commonest cause of magnesium deficiency is chronic alcoholism. The exact mechanism underlying this development is not known, however. Upon withdrawal of ethanol following long-term heavy consumption, the metabolic acidosis is replaced by respiratory alkalosis,[68] the seizure threshold is lowered and the signs and symptoms of magnesium deficiency become apparent, often culminating in grand mal seizures and even *status epilepticus*.

The concentration of magnesium in the CNS is normally high and it is a necessary cofactor in the operation of the magnesium-dependent Na^+/K^+—ATPase active transport system (the sodium-potassium pump, see above, figure 5). Ethanol at first inhibits the activity of Na^+/K^+—dependent ATPase probably because of its initial stimulatory effect upon central acetylcholine release. Acetylcholine inhibits the activity of Na^+/K^+—ATPase and the initial stimulation of acetylcholine release from central cholinergic neurons due to alcohol probably accounts at least partly for the early inhibition of the sodium-potassium pump. The subsequent depression of CNS acetylcholine release due to ethanol and the consequent inhibitory release of Na^+/K^+—ATPase may be responsible for the increased ATPase activity associated with chronic ethanol intake.

The role of the condensation products of amine neurotransmitters and their aldehyde metabolites due to the competetive inhibition by alcohol and acetaldehyde on their respective oxidases and reductases has already been discussed. A number of investigators have suggested that these THIQ's and beta-carbolines, some of which are on the biosynthetic pathway to morphine and codeine, may play a role in the development of the ethanol withdrawal syndrome. These condensates probably are not of major significance in the generation of this syndrome and the abstinence phenomena seen in ethanol withdrawal are quite different from those seen in opiate withdrawal. Nevertheless, there is evidence that these products, and in particular tetrahydropapaveroline, mediate some components of the ethanol withdrawal response.

Finally, a brief review of the several models of the pathogenesis of the ethanol withdrawal syndrome is appropriate at this point.[69]

(1) The *disturbed adaptation* model of H. Kalant and colleagues is based

---

[68]In uncompensated metabolic acidosis magnesium, along with other cation species, remains largely in the plasma compartment, and the manifestations of hypomagnesemia do not appear (muscle tremors, agitation, mental depression, hallucinations, delirium and epileptiform convulsions). In the presence of significant ethanol concentrations the acidosis is maintained, despite the body's attempts to reestablish normal acid-base balances by means of hyperventillation (see Light 1985), because of the continued generation of reducing equivalents from the oxidation of ethanol and acetaldehyde. Upon cessation of ethanol intake, however, hyperventillation soon restores blood pH to more normal values (the so-called "alkalosis" is a relative term in this context), the magnesium ions move *en masse* into the cellular compartment and become depleted in the plasma, and the signs and symptoms of magnesium deficiency, including lowered seizure threshold, occur.

[69]Taken largely from Feuerlein (1980).

upon the idea that the chronic intake of many addictive-prone drugs leads to adaptive changes in neurophysiological function which compensate for the effects of the drug and result in tolerance to the drug's effects, and which result in an overshoot response when the drug is withdrawn, thus giving rise to physical dependency. The mechanism of neural membrane hyperrigidity in response to chronic ethanol challenge described by Rottenburg *et al.* (1981) [see above, pages 96 to 101] as the major dynamic in the development of pharmacological tolerance and dependency is an elegant extension of the disturbed adaptation hypothesis. The suggestion that the intrusion of REM sleep resulting from rebound overshoot into the wakeful state is involved in alcoholic hallucinosis is another version of this model. It has also been proposed that a similar suppression of cAMP levels in second-messenger neurotransmitter systems during ethanol administration and subsequent rebound from inhibitory release when ethanol is withdrawn may also be implicated in the pathogenesis of withdrawal reactions, not only in the case of ethanol but also with many other addictive agents.

(2) The model of *electrolyte imbalance*, especially in disturbances in magnesium balance, in the generation of withdrawal manifestations has been previously discussed.

(3) The suggestion that delirium tremens and other severe withdrawal states may be a manifestation of "hepatic coma en miniature" (see Light 1985) were recently advanced in Germany (Feuerlein 1980). However, the EEG patterns characteristic of hepatic coma are not present in delerium tremens.

(4) The so-called *kindling model* of G. V. Doddard and R. M. Douglas has been recently applied to the ethanol withdrawal syndrome by J. C. Ballenger and R. M. Post (*in* Feuerlein 1980). This model proposes that frequent brain stimuli too low to produce any significant behavioral or EEG responses by themselves can induce progressively greater responses when summed over time, and particularly if they activate the limbic system. This is known as the *kindling effect*. It is proposed that repeated withdrawal episodes in chronic alcoholics act as kindling stimuli upon the limbic, hypothalamic and thalamic centers, and that the signs and symptoms of increasingly severe withdrawal states result from cumulative and progressive neurophysiological changes deriving from a cumulative, kindling process. This model suggests that ethanol withdrawal not only occurs upon termination of a drinking bout, but also approximately every 24 hours or so as the addict sleeps. The proponents of this theory

note that 24 hours is the optimal kindling interval in laboratory animals leading up to a seizurelike cumulative reaction to increasing EEG stimulatory kindling stages.

SUMMARY

Depression is associated with deficits in the levels and/or activity of the neurotransmitters norepinephrine and serotonin, although cholinergic systems also appear to be involved. This is now clearly established and is the accepted model among mainstream psychiatrists. Until recently depression was thought to fall into two distinct categories: endogenous depression, considered to represent essentially a biological disorder which could be effectively treated with antidepressant medications or electroconvulsive therapy, and reactive depression, thought to be largely psychogenic in origin which does not respond to chemical treatment. Recent clinical experience clearly shows, however, that depressive disorders appear to fall along a continuum and nearly always respond favorably to adequate doses of antidepressant medications given for sufficient periods. All clinical depression is now thought to involve genetic factors, although co-existing neurotic traits may also be present.

Depressions may be either unipolar or bipolar. Unipolar depressions involve one or more episodes of depression, with no manic or hypomanic manifestations. Such depressions may be confined to a single episode, or they may be recurrent or chronic. Recurrent depressive periods tend to eventually become chronic, at which point they may be referred to as chronic dysthymic disorder. Dysthymic disorder is considered to be a minor variant of major depressive disorder, and both respond well to antidepressant medications.

Bipolar disorder is diagnosed whenever a manic or hypomanic event occurs, and some authorities regard bipolar and unipolar depression as two fundamentally different states. However, unipolar depression often becomes bipolar disorder and other clinicians consider them to be two different manifestations of one basic psychiatric illness. Mania is the exact opposite of depression, and it reflects an excessive activity of norepinephrine in the brain. Both mania and severe depression can be very dangerous; manic patients have been known to kill others while in agitated states and depressives are all too likely to attempt or commit suicide. Bipolar swings between mania and depression have given rise to the term manic-depressive psychosis. Cyclothymic personality represents a minor variant, that is a less severe presentation, of manic-depressive disorder. Depressions can present as either psychomotor retardation or agitation, the former perhaps reflecting a norepinephrine deficit and the latter possibly involving inhibited serotoninergic activity. Depressive spectrum disorder refers to any depressive state in a person from a family in which alcoholism or sociopathy is also present in one or more family members.

Serotonin deficiency releases the normal inhibition of the amygdala, a portion of the limbic system involved in the conscious experience of emotion. This inhibition is equivalent to an indirect stimulation of the amygdala, resulting not only in psychic stress, anxiety and depression, but also to increased release of hydrocortisol from the adrenal glands. This compounds the emotional stress, leads to hypoglycemia and stimulates the release of tryptophan pyrrolase in the liver. This enzyme accelerates the breakdown of tryptophan, depriving the brain of this necessary precursor from which to synthesize serotonin. Thus serotonin is depleted still further, exacerbating the previously existing depression. Serotonin unavailability also decreases the inhibitory action of the raphe nuclei upon the R.A.S., leading to cortical hyperactivity, agitation and insomnia.

Serotonin deficiency has multiple and often contradictory effects upon the CNS. Serotoninergic pathways frequently possess feedback inhibitory loops. Thus the firing of a serotoninergic neuron with a collateral connection to an inhibitory interneuron, may paradoxically inhibit the same neuron which initiated the activity. Reduced levels of brain serotonin on the one hand release the inhibition of the raphe nuclei upon the R.A.S., indirectly stimulating it into spontaneous arousal. But the reduction in feedback inhibition may paradoxically enhance raphe activity, leading to a greater turnover rate for serotonin, which may in turn produce still greater serotonin deficit.

Chronic ethanol administration to laboratory animals results in lowered tryptophan pyrrolase in the brain (but acute ethanol administration increases the activity of this enzyme in the liver). Moreover, persons with high tonic arousal associated with R.A.S. hyperactivity show a marked decrease in such arousal after ethanol intake, and this is associated with the experience of pleasure. Alcohol exerts a general fluidizing effect upon neural membranes and multisynaptic, "reverberating" neuronal networks like the cerebral cortex, cerebellum and reticular formation are more profoundly affected than other systems. Depressed alcoholics typically display poor filtering or repressive competence which is very likely associated with reticular formation dysfunction in which serotonin deficiency may play an important role.

Low doses of ethanol facilitates neuronal activity by inhibiting the sodium-potassium pump, thus decreasing membrane polarity, and the early effects of slight membrane fluidization increase its permeability to sodium ions. The ensuing stimulation of the R.A.S. produces both excitatory and inhibitory effects: arousal is enhanced and anxiety due to psychonoxious material intruded into conscious awareness tends to be diminished. With increasing alcohol consumption, the initial slight stimulatory effect upon neural membranes is soon replaced by a much stronger depressant effect. The higher cortical regions of the brain with their complex reverberating neuronal networks are the first to be affected, and as they become depressed, the inhibitory function they exert upon lower centers is diminished. As the limbic system becomes disinhibited, labile emotions may spill over into conscious awareness. The contributes to the "paradoxical excitement" and social conviviality commonly observed as individuals become increasingly sedated by depressant drugs like alcohol, barbiturates, and anaesthetic gases used to induce surgical coma.

As drinking progresses, the depressant effect of the drug completely overrides any initial stimulatory effect it may exert. And cortical disinhibition permits ever deeper levels of emotional material to surge into "consciousness." But the corresponding decrease in awareness due to neocortical suppression more than compensates for "censorship-failure anxiety" resulting from intrusive psychonoxious material from the subconscious, and the bottom line for alcoholics is always blessed escape from the intense and constant interpersonal anxiety due to failure of both physiological and psychological repressive mechanisms.

Alcohol completely relieves such tension in alcoholic individuals. Although it promotes conviviality and relaxation in normal persons, they simply do not experience the complete relief from tension that alcohol appears to provide alcoholics. Alcoholics typically exhibit a poorly developed alpha brainwave pattern and this is associated with high tonic arousal, stress and dysphoria. In such individuals alcohol immediately produces a strong and stable alpha-pattern which is associated with a sense of serenity and well-being. And these effects persist long after all alcohol has been cleared from the body. The distinctive brainwave pattern seen in alcoholics is also exhibited by 40% or so of their male offspring—about the same proportion of children who later on manifest alcoholism themselves. These presumedly prealcoholic boys show the same poor alpha-rhythms seen in their alcoholic fathers, and this pre-dates any contact on their part with alcohol. And these children showed exactly the same response as their fathers when they were experimentally given alcohol! Chronic high tonic arousal and dysphoria so commonly experienced by alcoholically predisposed persons is readily alleviated by alcohol. These individuals feel better within themselves and in the context of interpersonal relationships; they develop a pattern of self-medicating with alcohol, and the very positive results they obtain rein-force their developing reliance upon the drug, and the addictive spiral is underway.

The first effective pharmacological agents used to treat depressive disorders were the MAO Inhibitors or MAOI's. These drugs inhibit the action of MAO. Thus, more of the deficient neurotransmitter tends to remain in the synaptic cleft for a longer period. More postsynaptic receptors are activated and the general effect is to produce neuronal responses commensurate with a greater concentration or higher activity of the neurotransmitter. But these agents also inhibit the activity of several liver enzymes and they potentiate the action of biogenic amines such as tyramine. If certain tyramine-containing foods are eaten while MAOI's are simultaneously administered, a very severe and even fatal hypertensive crisis may be precipitated.

The second class of antidepressant medications to appear are the so-called tricyclic antidepressants (TCA's). These are closely related to the anti-psychotic drugs known as phenothiazines, and like the latter they block the presynaptic reuptake of specific neurotransmitters as well as blockading postsynaptic receptor sites. In the case of the phenothiazines, the blockade of postsynaptic dopamine receptors is much greater than the inhibition of presynaptic reuptake. Thus, the major effect is to inhibit the activity of dopamine. Since schizophrenia is correlated with excessive dopaminergic activity in the thalamus and corpus striatum, the phenothiazines are useful in treating the more severe aspects of this disorder. The TCA's, however, block the presynaptic reuptake of norepinephrine, serotonin, or both, depending upon the specific medi-cation, to a much greater degree than they blockade the postsynaptic receptors. Their general effect, therefore, is to enhance the activity of those neurotransmitters, thereby compensating for the deficit. TCA's secondarily inhibit the action of phosphodiesterase which normally inactivates cAMP. Because serotonin and norepinephrine operate via a two-messenger system, these medications also cause the cAMP that is produced to remain active for a greater period, thus adding to the overall effect of neurotransmitter enhancement.

These drugs are very useful in treating depression and, if an adequate blood concentration can be developed and maintained for a sufficiently long period, usually three or four weeks, nearly all depressions can be alleviated. Despite statements in the literature to the contrary, antidepressant drugs are equally effective in treating both so-called "endogenous" and "reactive" or "neurotic" depressions. Clinical failures are almost always due to failure to obtain adequate blood levels of the medication and/or to maintain therapy long enough to get a clinical response. Because these drugs take several weeks to become effective (for reasons that are not understood) and very unpleasant side-effects appear almost immediately, patients initially feel even more uncomfortable on these medications. Thus, both the patient and the physician with little experience in using these agents tend to discontinue them prematurely. With continued therapy the worst aspects of the side-effects usually disappear.

Mania, generally regarded as resulting from excessive norepinephrine activity is typically treated with lithium salts. These agents enhance the presynaptic reuptake of norepinephrine, and this treatment is also very effective in treating bipolar disorder, sometimes in conjunction with TCA therapy. Lithium, however, is quite toxic and careful monitoring of the patient is usually necessary at first.

As previously stated, ethanol inhibits the sodium-potassium pump by interfering with ATPase. This diminishes the rate at which outward-leaking K^+ are returned to the intracellular medium. This reduces the resting potential of the membrane and the ensuing depolarization facilitates Na^+ permeability within the membrane and augments the generation of nervous activity. By packing into the phospholipid bilayer and increasing membrane fluidity, ethanol also increases the tendency for synaptic vesicles to fuse with the presynaptic membrane of the axon terminals. This results in elevated spontaneous release of neurotransmitters into the synaptic cleft, stimulating enhanced postsynaptic receptor activation. Ethanol-induced neural facilitation may therefore play a role in the "paradoxical" excitement seen in the early stages of intoxication. Such early facilitation of nervous transmission is soon overcome by the depressant effects of membrane fluidization as alcohol consumption continues, however. Cortical depression and inhibitory release of lower brain centers result in spontaneous surfacing of normally repressed emotions, resulting in an artificial social conviviality, and is the major factor underlying paradoxical excitement.

Ethanol is both polar and nonpolar. It is much more water soluble than lipid soluble and is readily distributed to all body water compartments. But because it is lipid soluble, it readily packs into the lipid portions of cell membranes, including nerve cells. Short-chain alcohols like ethanol are confined to the surface layer of membranes, with the ethyl groups embedded in the fatty acid moiety of the phospholipid double layer. The polar –OH groups project into the water fraction, however, and they probably interact electrostatically with the charged residues of the integral proteins. By packing into the membrane ethanol expands its volume, increasing membrane fluidity and distorting its architecture, causing the embedded proteins to malfunction.

Membrane fluidity is controlled by the number of unsaturated carbon atoms in the fatty acid tails of the phospholipids. Double bonds distort the orderly arrangement of the fatty acid tails. The presence of cholesterol molecules, however, counters this effect by forming stable complexes with the double carbon bonds. As membrane fluidity increases increased lateral motion of the component proteins is permitted. This increased lateral motion may cause decoupling of receptor-enzyme complexes such as those in two-messenger systems involving adenylate cyclase. Although the primary receptors may be activated by neurotransmitters, therefore, decoupling may prevent the sequence necessary to activate ionic channels.

Neural membranes respond to a chronic ethanol challenge by becoming more rigid—that is, less fluid. This occurs by decreasing the number of unsaturated carbon atoms in the fatty acid tails of the phospholipids. This presumably occurs by altering the protein components, which in turn influence the fatty acid sequences and thus the phospholipids of the bilayer. In addition, the cholesterol content of the membranes is greatly increased, thus stabilizing those double bonds which remain. This increases the membrane's tolerance to the fluidizing effects of alcohol, and more of the drug is required to achieve the desired effect. This process continues with continued alcohol intake and ultimately, with years of chronic alcohol abuse, the membranes can become so rigid that they can only function at all normally in the presence of the drug. Pharmacodynamic tolerance has now become physical dependence.

Biogenic amine neurotransmitters are broken down and inactivated by

MAO and COMT (5-HIOMT in the case of serotonin) into their alde-hyde intermediates. These aldehydes are then oxidized by aldehyde dehydrogenase into their corresponding acids or reduced by alcohol dehydrogenase into their alcohols. Such oxidation reactions require the reduction of NAD^+ into NADH plus H^+. And the corresponding reduc-tions require the oxidation of NADH plus H^+ into NAD^+.

The saturation of aldehyde dehydrogenase by acetaldehyde resulting from ethanol oxidation and the lack of oxidized NAD^+ effectively pre-vent amine aldehydes from being oxidized into their corresponding acids. And although the abundance of reduced NADH plus free hydro-gen ions would tend to shift the reaction in favor of reducing amine aldehydes into their alcohols, the complete saturation of alcohol dehy-drogenase by ethanol prevent this reaction as well. Thus amine alde-hydes tend to build up in the brain. Amine compounds (R–NH) and carbonyl compounds (R–HC=O) tend to undergo spontaneous non-enzymatic condensation reactions to form Schiff's bases (R–N=C–R). If the starting amino compound is a phenylethylamine such as dopamine, the condensation products thus formed will be tetrahydroisoquinolines or THIQ's. If the starting amino compounds are indolethylamines such as serotonin, the resulting condensation products will be tetrahydro-beta-carbolines.

These compounds interact with neurotransmitter functions in several ways. THIQ's compete with catecholamines (such as dopamine and norepinephrine) for presynaptic transport sites and for presynaptic stor-age vesicles. Because of this they competetively block the presynaptic reuptake of catecholamines and are preferentially taken up by the presynaptic storage vesicles. They thus exclude the normal transmitter substances from the synapse and interact with catacholaminergic post-synaptic receptors, acting as false transmitters. They also function as MAO inhibitors and this, together with their blockage of presynaptic catecholamine reuptake result in a buildup of both dopamine and norepinephrine. This produces an increase in the release of these neurotransmitters into the synaptic cleft. The buildup of catecholamine residues also increases the amount of amino compound involved in condensation reactions to form THIQ's. Because THIQ's inhibit the action of tyrosine hydroxylase, the synthesis of dopamine and norepi-nephrine is impeded. Together with the enhanced release of these catecholamines into the synaptic cleft, this results in depletion of these transmitters. THIQ's also cause a number of ultrastructural changes in adrenegric nerve terminals and associated Schwann cells.

Injections of THIQ's into the brains of normally ethanol-aversive rats produces greatly increased consumption of ethanol over that of control animals. The treated rats drink to the point of gross motor incapacitation and even physical withdrawal, and this continues for many months following treatment. Such studies present intriguing possibilities for the role these substances might play in the addictive process, and they are compounds occurring in the synthesis of morphine in the opium poppy. Nevertheless, most investigators believe that THIQ's play only a minor role in the etiology of alcoholism.

Ethanol's effect upon neurotransmitter release is complex and often contradictory. It has a biphasic effect upon acetylcholine and the catecholamines, both increasing and decreasing their release from synaptic terminals and their activity upon postsynaptic receptors. Similar effects of ethanol upon GABA activity have been reported, and it variously increases, decreases or has no effect at all upon GABA activity. Part of the confusion almost certainly results from the biphasic effect alcohol has upon nervous excitation, with low doses facilitating and higher doses impeding the production of nervous impulses.

Alcohol dehydrogenase is necessary to the metabolism of vitamin A and the production of rhodopsin necessary to vision. It is also vital to the production of testosterone. As a result, nightblindness reflecting avita-minosis A, and effeminization and sterility in males, are common signs of chronic alcoholism.

Both acute and chronic alcohol administration decrease the brain's capacity for protein synthesis, which contrasts markedly with the increase in protein synthesis exhibited by the liver in response to ethanol. The former phenomenon appears to be due to disruption of the enzymes by which tRNA molecules become "charged" with their specific amino acid and impaired functioning of the polyribosomal factories where proteins are synthesized. Increased protein synthesis in the liver in response to alcohol appears to be due to proliferation of the endoplasmic reticulum and Golgi apparatus which are involved in protein export from the cells (see Light 1985 for a discussion of this).

Small humps of tissue known as dendritic spines spontaneously form and dissipate over the surface of neuronal dendrites. When present they form ephemeral synapses with the axon terminals of other neurons. If one should happen to be utilized during the transmission of a nervous signal, that particular synapse will become more durable and tend to persist. If such pathways are used several times during the reinforcement of information processing, the synapses become very persistent. Reinforced material is thus associated with a permanent change in the actual structure of the brain, and it can supersede previously recorded information.

Learning and memory involve three major processes: (1) immediate memory is the registration and storage of information for only a few seconds: (2) this information is then transferred into short-term memory which lasts for a few minutes to several hours; short-term memory takes place largely in the thalamus and hippocampus and it involves electro-physiological changes in the neuronal units participating; (3) long-term memory is the consolidation and permanent storage of information transferred from the short-term memory; it involves alterations in mRNA and in the polypeptides synthesized from that mRNA. Unlike short-term memory traces, long-term memory is contained throughout the entire cerebral cortex. Because learning and memory appear to require the synthesis of specific proteins, the implications of ethanol-induced impairment of protein synthesis would seem to be clear.

Destruction to the mammillary bodies and hippocampus brought about by alcohol-induced thiamine deficiency coupled with the direct cytotoxic effects of chronic alcohol abuse result in the severe neurological impairment known as Wernicke-Korsakoff syndrome. Massive bilateral hippocampal destruction prevents the short-term memory system from retaining information long enough for it to be incorporated into long-term memory. Both immediate and long-term memories tend to remain more or less intact, but afflicted individuals cannot remember conversations that took place an hour or so before or what they had for breakfast or even if they had breakfast. Lesions in the mammillary bodies typically produce an apathetic and mild-mannered individual in a previously violent sociopath. Thiamine deficiency alone cannot produce Wernicke-Korsakoff-stage decompensation, and chronic ethanol abuse appears to be necessary in the etiology of this disorder.

Chronic ethanol administration produces learning impairment in laboratory animals which is associated with alterations in dendrite morphology and the number of neurons in the hippocampus and cerebellum. The number of dendritic spines is also significantly reduced in these regions.

CAT scans of the brains of chronic alcoholics reveals massive tissue atrophy and ventricular enlargement. These abnormalities are found in both young and older alcoholics, and these changes do not appear to revert back to normal with long-standing abstinence from alcohol (a year or more). These deficits appear to result from ethanol abuse itself and not from any previously existing neurological states. The degenerative changes seen in the brains of alcoholics are very similar to those of Alzheimer's disease due to aging, and several authors have suggested that alcohol abuse may be a contributing factor in some cases.

Hepatic encephalopathy develops from ammonia buildup in the brain due to gross liver failure and the impairment of hepatic detoxification processes. Peripheral polyneuropathy results from direct tissue damage due to alcohol as well as from massive loss of vitamins B-complex.

Normal sleep consists of two phases: REM or rapid eye movement sleep associated with dreaming and non-REM sleep. Ethanol decreases sleep latency, or the time one takes to fall asleep after going to bed. It also significantly decreases the amount of REM sleep, as do many other hypnotic drugs, and this effect occurs with even moderate doses of alcohol (blood-alcohol levels of 0.5 percent or less). Greater alcohol consumption correspondingly depresses REM sleep even more, and when alcohol is discontinued a rebound phenomenon is usually observed characterized by increased REM sleep time for several nights thereafter. REM sleep rebound occurs with most drugs which produce tolerance and dependence. Even alcoholics abstinent for three weeks show more REM sleep than do age-matched controls, and they exhibit more general arousal than controls. Several studies suggest that such sleep abnormalities persist for at least one or two and maybe even as long as four years in abstinent alcoholics. The sleep patterns of such persons is similar to that seen in elderly people.

The relationship between depression and alcoholism is clearly established. The agitated depression so commonly seen among alcoholic males may reflect serotonin insufficiency and a corresponding inhibitory release of the R.A.S., resulting in insomnia, restlessness, irritability, resentment, anxiety, frequent emotional outbursts and chronic dysphoria. Ethanol is known to potentiate the effects of serotonin in laboratory animals. And administration of 5-hydroxytryptophan to dry alcoholics greatly alleviates their insomnia. Melatonin, which is derived from serotonin, is also necessary to proper sleep patterns, and there is evidence that serotonin deficiency causes an increase in alcohol consumption in rats.

The ethanol-withdrawal syndrome is divided into three stages of increasing severity:

(1) First-phase withdrawal—reflects mild to moderate physical dependence and occurs generally eight to twenty-four hours after cessation of drinking; it is characterized by psychomotor agitation and tremors, anxiety, muscular weakness, nausea, and anorexia. These responses are immediately alleviated by ethanol intake and this often leads to morning (matutinal) drinking.

(2) Second-phase withdrawal—reflects moderate to severe physical dependence and with continued abstinence from ethanol generally occurs twelve to twenty-four hours following the onset of first-phase withdrawal; it is characterized by severe tremor, cramps, sweating, a rise in body temperature, diarrhea, severe nausea and vomiting, rapid pulse, hypertension and rapid breathing accompanied by a shift from ethanol-induced metabolic acidosis to respiratory alkalosis.

(3) Third-phase withdrawal—delirium tremens, reflecting extreme physical dependence. This life-threatening syndrome appears two to four days following the cessation of drinking, and the signs and symptoms of first- and second-phase withdrawal stages are continued into this phase. There may be extreme confusion and disorientation, agitation and panic, illusions and hallucinations, severe shakes along with muscular spasms, seizures and even *status epilepticus*, and mortality rates of 15 percent to more than 50 percent.

Factor 1 (first-phase) reactions derive from dysfunctions of cortical and sensory nerve pathways. Factor 2 (second-phase) reactions are thought to derive from disturbances in limbic system function. Factor 3 (third-phase) reactions are thought to derive from disturbances in brainstem function, including the cerebellum. All three factors can occur while alcohol is still being consumed.

Psychological stress appears to potentiate seizure activity during severe ethanol withdrawal, and constant, but reduced lighting, music and the avoidance of uniformed police officers on the detox ward reduce the incidence and severity of such seizures. American black males show a very high frequency of alcoholic hallucinosis relative to other ethnic and racial groups. This may be in part due to the fact that they are commonly seen in hospital emergency wards which are dominated by white authority figures. Psychological stress is known to potentiate the effects of heroin overdoses, and most fatal overdose outcomes occur when the patient finds himself in an unaccustomed environmental setting.

Alcoholic hallucinations may represent intrusions of dreams into the wakeful state of consciousness, perhaps associated with alcohol-induced REM sleep rebound. Spillover of dream material into consciousness has also been proposed for schizophreniform hallucinations. This idea has been criticized by other investigators, however.

Ethanol and other sedative-hypnotic agents raise the seizure threshold and confer protection against convulsions. There appears to be a rebound effect when the drugs are withdrawn, however, and the seizure threshold is temporarily lowered. A number of factors resulting from chronic alcohol abuse appear to play a facilitating role in the genesis of alcoholic seizures, including: hypoglycemia, magnesium deficiency and electrolyte imbalance resulting from ethanol-induced lactic- and ketoacidosis and malabsorbtion, and even the accumulation of THIQ's due to disordered biogenic amine metabolism resulting from long-term alcohol abuse.

The hyperrigid adaptation of neural membranes in response to sustained ethanol challenge is known to be involved in the development of physical tolerance and dependency. This is an example of the disturbed adaptation model of the development of withdrawal syndrome. It has also been suggested that delirium tremens and other severe withdrawal phenomena may represent "hepatic coma en miniature." And finally, the so-called kindling model of alcohol withdrawal postulates that continued brain responses to alcohol withdrawal which are in themselves too low to produce overt behavioral or EEG patterns may accumulate over time to a critical threshold where a seizure response finally does occur. This kindling effect is thought to act upon the hypothalamic and limbic centers. This model suggests that ethanol withdrawal not only occurs upon termination of a drinking bout, but also approximately every twenty-four hours as the alcoholic sleeps.

BIBLIOGRAPHY

Abu Murad, C., Begg, S. J., Griffiths, P. J., and Littleton, J. M.: Hepatic triglyceride accumulation and the ethanol physical withdrawal syndrome in mice. *British Journal of Experimental Pathology 58:* 606–615, 1977.

Becker, C. E., Roe, R. L., and Scott, R. A.: *Alcohol as a Drug: A Curriculum on Pharmacology, Neurology and Toxicology.* Baltimore: Williams & Wilkins, 1974.

Berry, M. S., and Pentreath, V. W.: The neurophysiology of alcohol. In Sandler, M. (Ed.): *Psychopharmacology of Alcohol.* New York: Raven Press, 1980, pp. 43–72.

Bowman, W. C., and Rand, M. J.: *Textbook of Pharmacology* (second edition). Oxford: Blackwell Scientific Publications, 1980.

Butters, N., and Cermak, L. S.: *Alcoholic Korsakoff's Syndrome: An Information-Processing Approach to Amnesia.* New York: Academic Press, 1980.

Calvin, W. H., and Ojemann, G. A.: *Inside the Brain.* New York: New American Library (Mentor), 1980.

Carlsson, A., and Lindqvist, M.: Antidepressants and brain monamine synthesis. *Journal of Neural Transmission 43:* 73, 1978.

Christensen, E. L., and Higgins, J. J.: Effect of acute and chronic administration of ethanol on the redox states of brain and liver. In Machrowicz, E., and Noble, E. P. (Eds.): *Biochemistry and Pharmacology of Ethanol.* New York: Plenum Press, 1979, vol. 1, pp. 191–247.

Cohen, G.: Interaction of catecholemines with acetaldehyde to form tetrahydroisoquinoline neurotransmitters. In Sharp, C. W., and Abood, L. G. (Eds.): *Progress in Clinical and Biological Research.* New York; Alan R. Liss, Inc., 1979, pp. 73–90.

Collins, M. A.: Monoamine condensations in human subjects. In Begleiter, H. (Ed.): *Biological Effects of Alcohol.* New York: Plenum Press, 1980, pp. 87–102.

Curran, M. L.: Brain waves may be alcoholism marker. *Family Practice News,* vol. 13, number 23, December 1–14, 1983, p. 34.

Cytryn, L., and McKnew, D. H., Jr.: Affective disorders. In *Comprehensive Textbook of Psychiatry/III.* Baltimore: Williams & Wilkins, 1980, vol. 3: 2798–2809.

The Diagram Group: *The Brain: A User's Manual.* New York: G. P. Putman's Sons, 1982.

Feuerlein, W.: Alcohol withdrawal syndromes. In Sandler, M. (Ed.): *Psychopharmacology of Alcohol.* New York: Raven Press, 1980, pp. 215–228.

Freund, G.: Diseases of the nervous system associated with alcoholism. In Tartar, R. E., and Sugarman, A. A. (Eds.): *Alcoholism: Interdisciplinary Approaches to an Enduring Problem.* Reading: Addison-Wesley Publishing Company, 1976, pp. 171–202.

Geller, I., and Purdy, R. H.: Interrelationship between ethanol consumption and circadian rhythm. In Machrowicz, E., and Noble, E. P. (Eds.): *Biochemistry and Pharmacology of Ethanol.* New York: Plenum Press, 1979, vol. 2: 453–465.

Golden, C. J., Graber, B., Blose, I., Berg, R., Coffman, J., and Bloch, S.: Difference in brain densities between chronic alcoholic and normal control patients. *Science 211:* 508–510, 1981.

Hökfelt, T., Johansson, O., and Goldstein, M.: Chemical anatomy of the brain. *Science 225:* 1326–1334, 1984.

Iversen, L. L.: The chemistry of the brain. *Scientific American 241* (3): 134–149, 1979.

Kaplan, H. I., and Sadock, B. J.: Neurophysiology of behaviour. In Kaplan, H. I., Freedman, A. M., and Sadock, B. J. (Eds.): *Comprehensive Textbook of Psychiatry/III* (3rd edition). Baltimore: Williams & Wilkins, 1980, vol. 1: pp. 189–211.

Klein, D. F., Gittelman, R., Quitkin, F., and Rifkin, A.: *Diagnosis and Drug Treatment of Psychiatric Disorders: Adults and Children* (2nd edition). Baltimore/London: Williams & Wilkins, 1980.

Kolata, G.: Clues to Alzheimer's disease emerge. *Science 210:* 941–942, 1983.

Lieber, C. S.: *Medical Disorders of Alcoholism: Pathogenesis and Treatment. Volume XXII. Major Problems in Internal Medicine.* Philadelphia: W. B. Saunders Company, 1982.

Light, W. J. H.: *Alcoholism: Its Natural History, Chemistry and General Metabolism.* Springfield: Charles C Thomas, 1985, volume 1.

Light, W. J. H.: *Psychodynamics of Alcoholism: A Current Synthesis.* Springfield: Charles C Thomas, in press, volume 3.

Light, W. J. H.: *Alcoholism and Women, Genetics, Fetal Development and Polydrug Abuse.* Springfield: Charles C Thomas, in press, volume 4.

Lishmann, W. A., Ron, M., and Acker, W.: Computed tomography of the brain and psychometric assessment of alcoholic patients—a British study. In Sandler, M. (Ed.): *Psychopharmacology of Alcohol.* New York: Raven Press, 1980, pp. 33–41.

Littleton, J. M.: The effects of alcohol on the cell membrane: a possible basis for tolerance and dependence. In Richter, D. (Ed.): *Addiction and Brain Damage.* London: Groom Helm, 1980, pp. 46–74.

Massarelli, R.: Effects of ethanol on the cholinergic system. In Machrowicz, E., and Noble, E. P. (Eds.): *Biochemistry and Pharmacology of Ethanol.* New York: Plenum Press, 1979, volume 2, pp. 223–240.

Melchior, C. L.: Long-lasting effects of tetrahydroisoquinolines. In Sandler, M. (Ed.): *Psychopharmacology of Alcohol.* New York: Raven Press, 1980, pp. 149–153.

Mendelson, W. B.: Pharmacologic and electrophysiologic effects of ethanol in relation to sleep. In Machrowicz, E., and Noble, E. P. (Eds.): *Biochemistry and Pharmacology of Ethanol.* New York: Plenum Press, 1979, volume 2, pp. 467–484.

Naranjo, C. A., Sellers, E. M., Roach, C. A., et al.: Zimelidine-induced variations in alcohol consumption by non-depressed heavy drinkers. *Clinical Pharmacology and Therapeutics 35:* 374–381, 1984.

Noble, E. P., and Tewari, S.: Metabolic aspects of alcoholism in the brain. In Lieber, C. S. (Ed.): *Metabolic Aspects of Alcoholism.* Baltimore: MTP (University Park Press), 1978, pp. 1–29.

O'Briant, R. G., and Lennard, H. L.: *Recovery From Alcoholism: A Social Treatment Model.* Springfield: Charles C Thomas, 1973.

Oswald, W., and Azevedo, I.: Chemical sympathectomy due to tetrahydroisoquinolines derived from adrenalin. In Begleiter, H. (Ed.): *Biological Effects of Alcoholism.* New York: Plenum Press, 1980, pp. 131–136.

Pollock, W. E., Volavka, J., Goodwin, D. W., Mednik, S. A., Gabrielli, W. F., Knop, J., and Schulsinger, F.: The EEG after alcohol administration in men at risk for alcoholism. *Archives of Geberal Psychiatry 40:* 857–861, 1983.

Reitz, R. C.: Effect of ethanol on carnitine acyltransferase. *Federal Proceedings 36:*331, 1977. [Abstract.]

Reitz, R. C.: Effect of ethanol on the intermediary metabolism of liver and brain. In Machrowicz,

E., and Noble, E. P. (Eds.): *Biochemistry and Pharmacology of Ethanol.* New York: Plenum Press, 1979, volume 1, pp. 353–382.

Restak, R. M.: *The Brain.* Toronto: Bantam Books, 1984.

Roach, M. K.: Changes in the activity of Na^+, K^+–ATPase during acute and chronic administration of ethanol. In Machrowicz, E., and Noble, E. P. (Eds.): *Biochemistry and Pharmacology of Ethanol.* New York: Plenum Press, 1979, volume 2, pp. 67–80.

Rottenburg, H., Waring, A., and Rubin, E.: Tolerance and cross-tolerance in chronic alcoholics: reduced membrane binding of ethanol and other drugs. *Science 213:*583–584, 1981.

Schramm, M., and Selinger, Z.: Message transmission: receptor controlled adenylate cyclase system. *Science 225:*1350–1356, 1984.

Schukit, M. A.: *Drug and Alcohol Abuse: A Clinical Guide to Diagnosis and Treatment.* New York; Plenum Press, 1979.

Seiden, L. S., and Dykstra, L. A.: *Psychopharmacology: A Biochemical and Behavioral Approach.* New York: Van Nostrand Reinhold Company, 1977.

Shaw, S., and Lieber, C. S.: Amino acids and ethanol. In Machrowicz, E., and Noble, E. P. (Eds.): *Biochemistry and Pharmacology of Ethanol.* New York: Plenum Press, 1979, volume 1, pp. 383–406.

Siegel, S., Hinson, R. E., Krank, M. D., and McCully, J.: Heroin "overdose" death: contribution of drug-associated environmental cues. *Science 216:*436–437, 1982.

Stevens, C. F.: The neuron. *Scientific American 241:*54–65, 1979.

Walker, D. W., Barnes, D. E., Riley, J. N., Hunter, B. E., and Zornetzer, S. F.: Neurotoxicity of chronic alcohol consumption: an animal model. In Sandler, M. (Ed.): *Psychopharmacology of Alcohol.* New York: Raven Press, 1980, pp. 17–31.

Warwick, R., and Williams, P. L.: *Gray's Anatomy* (35th British edition). Philadelphia: W. B. Saunders Company, 1973.

White, A., Handler, P., Smith, E. L., Hill, R. L., and Lehman, I. R.: *Principles of Biochemistry.* New York: McGraw-Hill Book Company, 1978.

INDEX

155

H

Haeckel, Ernst, 46
Hallucinations, association alcohol-induced REM
    sleep rebound and, 150
Handler, P., 31, 110, 153
Hepatic encephalopathy
    cause, 148
    toxic mechanism of, 123
Heroin
    effects environment on overdose, 132–133,
        149–150
        results studies of, 133
    opiate derivative, 31, 68
Higgins, J. J., 109, 151
Hill, R. L., 31, 110, 153
Hinsdill, Ronald D., xv
Hinson, R. E., 132, 133, 153
Hippocampus
    destruction of, 147
        cause, 147
    effects damage to, 58
    involvement in emotional control, 58
    origin of, 52
        diagram, 54, 56
Hoddes, 127
Hökfelt, T., 42, 152
Hordenine, source of, 103
Hormones
    definition, 68
    released by hypothalamus, 68–69
        oxytocin, 68–69
        vasopressin, 68–69
Hunter, B. E., 119, 120, 122, 153
Hydrocortisone (*see* Cortisol)
5-Hydroxytryptamine (*see* Serotonin)
Hyperkinesis, childhood (*see* Childhood
    hyperkinesis)
Hypoglycemia, due production hydrocortisol,
    78
Hypomania, treatment of, 93
Hypophysiotropic hormones, effects on pituitary,
    35, 37
Hypothalamus
    cholinoceptive neurons in, 45
    control of by limbic system, 72
    effect removal of, 57
    formation mammillary bodies, 55, 71
        diagram, 57
    formation pituitary gland, 71
        diagram, 57
    involvement in expressions of emotion,
        57, 71
    rage induced by, 56–57

I

Imipramine
    as tertiary amine, 90
    use to treat cataplexy, 80
Indole, 23, 24
    diagram, 24
    effects of, 23
Indolethylamine, condensation products of, 103
Insomnia
    cause of, 62
        interactions of naphe nuclei, diagram, 62
    early, due serotonin deficiency, 90–91
        treatment of, 91
    early versus terminal, 76–77
    melatonin deficit in, 86
        treatment of, 86
    production of, 62, 72
    psychological depression and, 62
    treatment of in dry alcoholics, 148
    with agitated depression, 78
Insulin, effect on amino acids, 62–63
Isoniazid
    effect on depression, 87
    inhibitors of monoamine oxidase, 87
Iversen, L. L., 21, 31, 152

J

Johansson, O., 42, 152

K

Kalant, H., 135
Kaplan, H. I., 79, 81, 152
Klein, D. F., 92, 93, 152
Knop, J., 84, 152
Kolata, G., 123, 152
Krank, M. D., 132, 133, 153

L

L-DOPA, conversi
    conversion to dopa decarboxylase, 23, 25
    formation of, 25, 26
        diagram, 24
    source of, 22–23
    treatment Parkinson's Disease using, 56
LSD-25, source of, 103–104
L-tryptophas, effects on sleep when added to
    serotonin, 127
Learning
    association with RNA, 117
    changes in S-100 and, 117